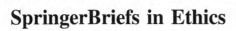

SpringerBriefs in Ethics

MW00397599

More information about this series at http://www.springer.com/series/10184

Jeffrey P. Spike · Rebecca Lunstroth

A Casebook
in Interprofessional Ethics

A Succinct Introduction to Ethics
for the Health Professions

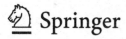 Springer

Jeffrey P. Spike
McGovern Center
The University of Texas Health Science
  Center at Houston, UTHealth
Houston, TX
USA

Rebecca Lunstroth
McGovern Center
The University of Texas Health Science
  Center at Houston, UTHealth
Houston, TX
USA

ISSN 2211-8101   ISSN 2211-811X   (electronic)
SpringerBriefs in Ethics
ISBN 978-3-319-23768-8   ISBN 978-3-319-23769-5   (eBook)
DOI 10.1007/978-3-319-23769-5

Library of Congress Control Number: 2015959909

Printed on acid-free paper

This Springer imprint is published by SpringerNature
The registered company is Springer International Publishing AG Switzerland

To my wife Elizabeth Spike, and to the lights of my life: Alexander Hume, Perry Spinoza, and Sophia Russell Spike, my three teenage children who are rapidly becoming unique and wonderful individuals.

Acknowledgments

It is important to acknowledge that this book is the result of a group project. In 2009, the President of The University of Texas Health Science Center-Houston gave financial support to faculty from all six professional schools to develop and enhance the ethics curriculum, the Campus-wide Ethics Program (or CWEP). The first three years were spent identifying core ethics topics essential to be introduced to all students, regardless of professional school. The result was a book entitled *The Brewsters*, which is required reading for first-year students in every degree program at all six of our schools: Medicine, Nursing, Public Health, Dentistry, Biomedical Sciences, and Informatics. (If you want to know more about *The Brewsters*, you can go to the Web site MeetTheBrewsters.com.) After that the CWEP turned to working on the newest challenge in ethics, interprofessional ethics. The cases in this book represent the work of the CWEP from 2012 to 2014.

I must particularly acknowledge the work of my colleagues in the McGovern Center for Humanities and Ethics at UT-Houston. First, our administrative assistants, Angela Polczynski, who helped arrange rooms, keep records, and maintain the group's pace over the years of monthly meetings, and Alma Rosas who helped keep track of many revisions of the manuscript, and second, Rebecca Lunstroth, J. D., the Assistant Director of the McGovern Center, and the co-director of the medical school and the school of biomedical science's ethics and professionalism courses. Rebecca took on the task of final editing of the cases in Chap. 6 of the book, making improvements to all of them. I also must acknowledge the support and encouragement of this project by the Director of the McGovern Center, Tom Cole.

One member of the Campus-wide faculty, Stephen Linder from the School of Public Health, provided some conceptual organization to the group process that was especially helpful to the group. His contributions led to his writing the first draft of chapter two, "Framing Interprofessional Ethics Cases." He deserves special acknowledgment as a co-author of that chapter.

viiiAcknowledgments

I also thank The Hastings Center for hosting me during the process of finishing the first five chapters of the book, and to my wife Elizabeth Spike, my research assistant Jennifer Bulcock, and Laura Haupt at The Hastings Center who read and helped edit those five chapters.

Contents

About the Senior Author and Editor

Jeffrey P. Spike Ph.D. is the Samuel Karff Professor in the McGovern Center for Humanities and Ethics at The University of Texas Health Science Center-Houston, and Director of the UTHealth Campus-wide Ethics Program.

Dr. Spike has been working full-time in medical education since receiving his Ph.D. in philosophy from The Johns Hopkins University in 1987. Dr. Spike is on the editorial board of Narrative Inquiry in Bioethics and is the co-editor of the clinical ethics cases in The American Journal of Bioethics. He has taught required medical school and public health courses on ethics and professionalism, as well as numerous elective courses. He also regularly lectures to medical school clerks and residents in Medicine, Pediatrics, Neurology, OB, and Psychiatry, and in General, Acute, Maxillofacial, and Maternal-Fetal Surgery.

Dr. Spike has started, been a member of, or chaired ethics committees at seven hospitals, a hospice, an insurance company, and a nursing home. Spike is also head of the clinical ethics affinity group of the American Society for Bioethics and Humanities, and for many years led their preconference workshop on advanced skills for clinical ethics consultation.

Spike has been on the curriculum committee at the three medical schools where he has taught, and published curriculum in MedEdPortal on professionalism and on using films and television shows as sources of rich narratives for teaching. He has written articles and facilitator guides to *The Doctor*, *Lorenzo's Oil*, *Dax's Case*, *Wit*, and an episode of *Scrubs*. His most recent adventure in making learning ethics more fun was co-authoring a book that intertwines a fictional story about healthcare providers with lessons about professionalism, clinical ethics, and research ethics. The book is entitled *"The Brewsters,"* and can be bought on iTunes.

Ways to Use This Book

This book is written in a style meant to be easily accessible to most students in the health sciences, whether beginning graduate-level students in medicine, dentistry, nursing, or public health or advanced undergraduate students preparing for graduate-level education in the health sciences (e.g., premed students or pre-health science students). It can be used as the primary text for a course or as an adjunct to a textbook. In particular, it is designed to be short enough and inexpensive enough that a teacher can assign it in addition to any one of the hundreds of standard textbooks in the health sciences whose ethics content is limited in focus to just one profession (medical ethics, nursing ethics, dental ethics, etc.). It is also designed to be a valuable addition to a course that is not primarily about ethics when the instructor wishes to have more than the usual one chapter on ethics included in so many of the survey textbooks used to introduce a health profession.

This book is also useful for professional development for working doctors, nurses, or social workers in a hospital. For example, a hospital seeking nursing magnet status could incorporate this into a series of interprofessional rounds and online discussions, to aid in their application. In particular, in the USA, where the number of bachelor-level registered nurses and master- and doctoral-level nurse practitioners has grown, recognizing their professional status is vital to having a good process. Though these interprofessional rounds can be invaluable, overcoming the inertia of separate professions can be difficult. Having a few chapters of a book to read and discuss together might provide the material needed to get members of different professions to come together in the same room and talk. That first step can be the most difficult, and so this simple use of the book might just turn out to be of great practical value.

There are also interdisciplinary fellowship programs, such as in palliative care, that are open to trainees from various professions. These programs obviously do not have the obstacles to overcome that many other programs face. However, an introduction to healthcare ethics that is designed to be profession-neutral could be a useful tool. Even in such open forums as interdisciplinary fellowship programs, there are often feelings of lack of recognition on the part of some members that might go unspoken, and a book of interprofessional ethics can help make explicit that the most important issues do not belong to any one group and are best handled by having representation from all the groups.

A quick aside on the meaning of interprofessional education: Some authors insist that the ideal is to have the trainees from different professions in the same room. At a certain level of training, this can be done and is worth the extra effort. Residents in OB-GYN could, for example, have ethics rounds with nurses in a master's degree program in woman's health or midwifery. But many other situations would not be so easy to arrange, largely because the students would be in different buildings at different times. In such cases, one might still try to arrange a single two- or three-hour module once a semester or once a year, with students broken down into small groups (usually defined as around six to eight students) with representation from two schools in each small group. But one must never make the best the enemy of the good; online education has become widely accepted and used in many settings and can be an effective way to have students from different schools share a reading and discuss a case together.

There is one other option to mention as a possible use of this text. This book can be used as a follow-up to a book titled *The Brewsters*, also written by Jeffrey Spike with members of the campus-wide ethics program. *The Brewsters* introduces ethics to students entering health professions using a narrative approach. It offers a story about a fictional family, enhancing the narrative approach even further by making it a "choose-your-own-adventure," that is, an interactive format. The format works by engaging the reader in the story as a participant, or moral agent, who faces decisions, makes choices, and then proceeds to discover the consequences. By using characters the students can identify with and putting them into realistic situations students might face, *The Brewsters* challenges students to wrestle intellectually with the kinds of issues they are likely to deal with in their chosen profession. (To find out more about *The Brewsters*, or to order a copy in paperback, go to MeetTheBrewsters.com. It is also available from Amazon and as an iTunes download.)

Whether this casebook is used along with another book on ethics in one particular profession or with a general introductory textbook to a profession, or for professional development, or as an adjunct to *The Brewsters*, its goals are the same: first, to show that ethics is an essential and inherent part of what it means to be a professional in health care and that learning ethical issues and how to deal with them in advance should be as important a part of the preparation to enter a field as learning how to start an IV or central line or how to assess the scientific validity of a statistical analysis of a large database. And second, while ethics in each of the health professions has made great progress, that progress has come one field at a time, and so this book intends to facilitate an appreciation that now is the time for a new approach: interprofessional ethics. It is not a change in what is ethical, as if the health professions had made any terrible blunders, but it is time for the health professions to recognize their interconnectivity and mutual dependence and for ethics to be recognized as the core discipline to bring them together, the glue, as it were, of interprofessional education.

A note about this book: This book is a collaborative effort of the Campus-wide Ethics Program at the University of Texas-Houston, an academic health science center. The director of the program, Jeffrey P. Spike, has taught in medical, nursing, biomedical science, and public health schools for twenty-five years. He organized the book and is a coauthor of all the chapters and cases. However, other CWEP faculty contributed to every chapter and case. The names and titles of the CWEP faculty members are listed below and again in the introduction to the cases in Chap. 6. The aim of this book was not primarily to propose a new claim about what ethics is or requires of healthcare professionals (although that may happen as well), but to present ethics in a way that makes it readily accessible, improves students' incorporation of ethical issues into their thinking, and helps them work collaboratively in teams in their current or future health profession.

Director:
Jeffrey P. Spike, Ph.D.

Medical School:
Eugene Boisaubin, M.D.
Nathan Carlin, Ph.D.

School of Dentistry:
Richard Bebermeyer, D.D.S., M.B.A.
Catherine Flaitz, D.D.S., M.S.

School of Nursing:
Joan Engebretson, Dr.P.H., R.N., AHN-BC
Dorothy Otto, M.S.N., Ed.D., R.N.
Cathy Rozmus, Ph.D., R.N.

School of Public Health:
Stephen Linder, Ph.D.
Cynthia Chappell, Ph.D.

School of Biomedical Informatics:
Jonathan Ishee, J.D., M.P.H., M.S., L.L.M

Graduate School of Biomedical Sciences:
William Seifert, Jr., Ph.D.
Rebecca Lunstroth, J.D., M.A.

Chapter 1
A Very Brief History of Health Care Ethics: Four Decades from the Golden Age of Bioethics to the Dawn of Interprofessional Ethics

An eighteen-month-old girl's death from dehydration in 2010 at Johns Hopkins Hospital in Baltimore provides a sobering example of the need for interprofessional ethics training. In a *New York Times* interview, Dr. Peter Pronovost, medical director of the Quality and Safety Research Group at the hospital, admitted, "We had dysfunctional teamwork because of an exceedingly hierarchal culture. When confrontations occurred, the problem was rarely framed in terms of what was best for the patient" (March 9, 2010). Lives are lost sometimes, in other words, on account of poor teamwork. Hence, promoting effective teamwork is an ethical imperative. Teaching a coherent and consistent clinical and research ethics framework that is shared by all professions, in an interprofessional setting, will allow bioethics to be more successfully integrated into the work of all health care professionals.[1]

The field of bioethics is evolving. This evolution, which yields new questions and opportunities for the health care field, can be observed in three stages of its development. The first stage, which one might call the Golden Age, was inaugurated when a few influential books identified a new terrain that came to be called "bioethics." To name only a few luminaries, authors such as Tom Beauchamp, Al Jonsen, Dan Callahan, Sam Gorovitz, Stephen Toulmin, Ruth Macklin, George Annas, Bob Veatch, Mary Warnock, Alex Capron, and Tris Englehardt identified the core topics, formulated principles and practices for addressing ethical dilemmas, and articulated the importance of secular bioethics in a pluralistic society. These early bioethicists mainly worked in bioethics centers, or "think tanks," such as the Kennedy Institute at Georgetown University and The Hastings Center in upstate New York.

This groundwork laid the foundations for bioethics institutes, journals, and emerging curricula in medical schools across the English-speaking world and, later, beyond. This Golden Age, which might be dated from the early 1970s through the 1980s, emerged on account, to a large extent, of embarrassing research scandals in history, scandals on which individuals such as Henry Beecher and Maurice

---

[1]The patient safety movement, and the concern to find ways to reduce errors was greatly stimulated by the publication of *To Err Is Human* by the Institute of Medicine, IOM, National Academy Press, 2000.

© The Author(s) 2016
J.P. Spike and R. Lunstroth, *A Casebook in Interprofessional Ethics*,
SpringerBriefs in Ethics, DOI 10.1007/978-3-319-23769-5_1

Pappworth first blew the whistle in the late 1960s.[2] Even their early warnings might have been ignored were it not for some scandals that occurred on the heels of the American civil rights movement.[3]

The second stage, what one might call the Silver Age, was inaugurated when bioethicists began to work more often in medical centers and began to enlarge the range of topics of interest to the field. The early work in the field could mostly be characterized as concerned with issues in internal medicine and, especially, end-of-life care (or as it was sometimes known, the right to die). However, from the mid-1980s through the 1990s, more attention came to bear on virtually every specialty from pediatrics to OB-GYN to surgery.

This stage also received an initial boost from public scandals, as political and ethical debates raged concerning a number of Baby Doe cases concerning whether to provide surgery to handicapped newborns, or select non-treatment as a humane alternative to allow a quick and peaceful death. Initial cases concerned babies with Down's syndrome, leading to rich discussions of the value of life of the disabled, and whether many in society, including many doctors, were undervaluing the lives of the disabled. These discussions included professionals in pediatrics and neonatology as well as surgery, enlarging the circle of professions and specialties recognizing the importance of clinical ethics in their decision-making process. Throughout this Silver Age, more and more physicians were receiving training in basic medical ethics in their medical education, and many subspecialties were identifying their own ethical concerns. Nursing, dentistry, and other health fields soon followed this same path.

The narrative of the Silver Age, then, centers on ethics first entering the internal practices of medicine more as a participant than an outsider and, simultaneously, extending the reach of bioethics beyond the profession of medicine to other health professions. These expansions in depth and breadth characterize the 1990s above all and continued until quite recently. Exemplars of this second age of bioethics include William Bartholome and Robert Weir in pediatrics, Laurence McCullough in OB-GYN and surgery, K.W.M. Fulford in psychiatry, David Ozar and Thomas Hasegawa in dentistry, and Sara Fry and Andrew Jameton in nursing. Also of note in this stage is that ethics cases and serious analysis of ethical issues in practice came more often to be published in medical journals, including specialty journals, and in journals of other health professions—not just in ethics journals.

It might appear that, since bioethics has now become incorporated into all of the health professional fields, there is little left to do other than to continue refining and deepening our analysis. While such refining and deepening will always need to be done, other developments in bioethics merit a revision in the narrative of bioethics. We believe an important third stage of bioethics is just beginning, a stage one might call the Bronze Age.

---

[2]Especially the Tuskegee study of untreated syphilis in African Americans.

[3]M.H. Pappworth, *Human Guinea Pigs*. Routledge and Kegan Paul, London, 1967. H. Beecher, "Ethics and Clinical Research," New Eng J Med, 274: 1354–1360.

What, then, constitutes the new material for this emerging age in bioethics? We suggest that it is interprofessional ethics. Consider that there might be an ethics for pediatrics as well as an ethics for nursing—what is one to do if they are in conflict? Shall we train our doctors and our nurses to believe that different courses of action are the right ones, leading to interprofessional conflict? Should we let the more powerful or well-funded disciplines always have the last say as to what is the best course of treatment, a recipe guaranteed to lead to moral distress for those who feel disempowered? These are rhetorical questions, meant to bring out the importance of the new questions we wish to add to the canon of values developed and promoted by bioethics (which we take to include clinical ethics and research ethics).

A couple examples of types of conflicts, as well as examples of specific cases, will spell out what we mean more clearly. The first type of conflict is *intra*professional but interdisciplinary. It is seen in cases where, for example, two doctors disagree about what to do when both are treating the same patient. For instance, an internist believes that the best plan involves pharmacological interventions, whereas a surgeon prefers surgical interventions. Another example might involve an anesthesiologist who recommends conscious sedation or a regional block over the preference of a surgeon for a general anesthetic. While traditional codes of professionalism might have insisted on the importance of never openly disagreeing with another doctor and of leaving the final decision to whoever is higher in the medical hierarchy, modern bioethics would see this prohibition as a violation of patient's rights and the traditional solution as an ethical failure.

Another type of conflict is *inter*professional. This arises in cases where health care professionals from different professions, such as doctors and nurses, disagree. Doctors and nurses, of course, must work together as a team, which is as important in a private office as in the hospital setting. Thus nursing ethics and medical ethics must be congruent if they are to encourage cooperation rather than ethical conflict. But the number of health professions that ought to be included is far more than just nursing and medicine: social work; the field of physician assistants; occupational, physical, radiation, and speech therapy; optometry; pharmacy; public health; dentistry; dental hygiene; health informatics; imaging technology; and numerous others need to have a voice.

This book is the first to address the need for a clearly interdisciplinary and interprofessional ethics. To make the point with dramatic flourish, we propose a third stage of development of bioethics wherein we would abolish (more accurately, transcend) the traditional categories of medical ethics and nursing ethics and dental ethics (and anesthesthiologcal ethics, surgical ethics, etc.).

Here is an example of an ordinary situation that demonstrates potential interprofessional conflict. A ninety-year-old patient comes into the hospital through the ER at night for shortness of breath. After admission, the patient tells the nurse some of her greatest fears and says that she would "never want to be intubated—no matter what." The nurse discusses this with her and tries to persuade her otherwise, but the patient is quite adamant. By morning, when the rest of the medical team finally sees her, she is obtunded, and no family can be found. The hope is that she will need to be on a ventilator for only three days and that a course of IV antibiotics will enable her to overcome her pneumonia and be weaned from the vent. The nurse, acting as a patient advocate (an important role according to nursing ethics) explains the patient's views to the team, but many members are skeptical. How should situations like these be handled? Which values, perspectives, and voices should be given the most weight? How, practically, does the team move forward? If the team intubates the patient, will this lead to a general devaluing of patient preferences in medical decision-making, for example, seeing geriatric patients as just too uninformed to be allowed to make important life-and-death decisions? And will that, in turn, undermine the input of nurses who accept the charge of being patient advocates, and create moral distress?

These types of conflicts must be anticipated during training. When one observes how many different professionals see each patient, one will see that these situations are not at all rare but, rather, daily occurrences. Most hospitalized patients will see a number of doctors and a number of nurses, and there will often be routinely scheduled team meetings with representatives of different professions to review cases. If we do not notice such conflicts more often, it may be because of our monocular bias, in other words, that we tend to see the perspective of the professional who called for an ethics consult, or the perspective of the attending because he or she is thought to be legally in charge. But any such narrow focus leads to oversimplifications of complex cases and ignores power imbalances. Extending bioethics to interprofessional approaches can help to equalize the different professional viewpoints and, in the process, bring a patient-centered perspective to the foreground.

The Bronze Age may someday also come to be seen as emerging out of, not any single scandal, but a type of crisis that has brought the need for a wider approach to our attention. It is the crisis over the mishandling of mistakes by health care providers and how to avoid them. The patient-safety movement is not usually thought of as primarily ethical, although the advice that we ought to be more honest about our mistakes certainly is. But we would argue that even the attempts to minimize error can be thought of as inherently ethical, a part of what could appropriately be called preventive ethics. That is a core lesson that the Johns Hopkins case (above) teaches, and is increasingly recognized as important in hospitals everywhere: the authoritarian model of one man (or woman) in charge led to increased risks.

The Bronze Age of bioethics, we suggest, should involve the teaching of consistent viewpoints across various professions so that our teaching improves—and does not unintentionally undermine—the relationships among team members. The intent is to help the team to perform more efficiently and effectively, as well as more ethically. What is needed, in other words, is an articulation of sets of interprofessional and dialogical principles, values, and practices that encourage genuine teamwork by all members of health care teams. The purpose is to be more patient-centered and to have all team members be more consciously aware that both the quality of health care and the satisfaction of patients will improve if they all share the same patient-centered ethics.

What is emerging in the field of bioethics is consistent with larger trends in the education of health professionals. In 1978, the World Health Organization first indicated that interprofessional education is an important component in the education of health professionals (Hoffman and Harnish 2007). The British have especially been leaders in recognizing the value of interprofessional ethics (Freeth 2007). Interprofessional practice has been defined as "a patient-centered, team-based approach to health care delivery that synergistically maximizes the strengths and skills of each contributing health professional" (Hoffman and Harnish 2007). Various studies have shown that interprofessional practice often leads to improved patient care and higher levels of work satisfaction (for a review of this literature, see Stone 2006).

Though there have been calls for more interprofessional education for years, there have been few efforts and even fewer successes. We believe that there are two primary reasons for this. First, the problem with interdisciplinary education outside of the clinical setting has been largely spatiotemporal: different schools have different schedules and many students (such as in nursing) have part- or full-time jobs in addition to their coursework or clinical hours. But the advent and burgeoning growth of web-based distance learning means that the impossible has become possible: we can now teach students from different schools the same material more or less simultaneously, and allow them to interact online using social media, discussion boards, blogs, wikis, and other methods.

Second, there has been resistance from each profession over the knowledge base it considers essential to its expertise. These "turf wars" can prevent each group from admitting that other groups have equally valuable knowledge to share. At its best, each profession identifies and uses its expertise in order to avoid border skirmishes. Dentists must respect hygienists' turf, and vice versa—similarly for doctors and nurses, ophthalmologists and optometrists, gastroenterologists and speech therapists. However, if one's view of one's expertise is expanded to include ethics, each profession might think its ethics gives it an authority over other professions' ethics; however no one profession should see ethics as uniquely part of their turf in such a way that it gives them the right to make decisions without the input of the other members of the team. Ethics, as a subject, must always be willing to move up one step in generality to allow a dialogue that includes other viewpoints or justifications.

Interprofessional ethics education, we believe, promises to be a vital approach that will overcome this resistance and promote interprofessional practice. There is no subject that is more fitting as the unifying focus for a team approach to the patient. Interprofessional ethics education will also prove to be an intellectual area of study in the field of bioethics worthy of pursuit in its own right. A group of scholars at the University of Colorado Health Sciences Center predicted the importance of interprofessional ethics education in an article describing their attempt to implement such teaching at their institution (Yarborough et al. 2000). They were, however, at the beginning of these efforts and had limited success (personal correspondence). We believe the time for the ascendance of this new paradigm is now.

We do not mean to suggest that bioethics has "figured everything out" and that the project of the Bronze Age of bioethics is to impose a universal set of standards or a packaged set of answers to various specialties and professions. Ethics, like every other subject of human knowledge, changes over time; it progresses. What we are suggesting, however, is that what is needed, and what is in fact emerging in bioethics, is a new stage of development invigorated by conscious attention to intra- and interprofessional dialogue. We are, in other words, realizing the importance of input from many professions, including scientific and professional fields as well as philosophy, before reaching a consensus. In our experience, some of the best educational venues in the hospital setting involve rounds with attending physicians, fellows, residents, nurses, and social workers working together on specific cases. Members of each of these professions have found that it is extremely valuable to hear the others' views while discussing a case around a conference table. Such educational experiences are not only interesting because they produce new kinds of knowledge for everyone involved, but also are a practical form of teambuilding through engaging in a dialogue with a common goal of reaching a consensus. But, to be honest, such rounds are rare and hard to institute. Each profession is more comfortable with its own, with people from a shared professional background. It is important for all professions to come to recognize this insularity is counterpro- ductive when it comes to ethics.

Our book of interprofessional cases is meant to help achieve this goal by pro- viding a common vocabulary to all students, across all the health professions, in order to improve communication and enhance understanding among the profes- sions. A natural and valuable side effect from this approach is to empower those who might see themselves as part of a less powerful profession to speak up as equal team members and to make those who might see themselves as members of a more powerful profession be more willing to see other members of the team as equal partners when it comes to identifying and dealing with ethical issues. The final goal of these interprofessional rounds, and the purpose of ethics, is to recognize and resolve professional differences fairly, and to thereby also create the space for patient-centered perspectives.

We are implementing a campus-wide ethics program at our own institution. The faculty at the McGovern Center for Humanities and Ethics at UTHealth (the aca- demic health science center of the University of Texas in Houston) and affiliated faculty from the six schools at UTHealth have developed the following interdis- ciplinary cases to be presented to students in existing classes and via online resources. Our intent is that students will read and respond to the cases, using assigned readings for guidance. Using online distance learning, they will be able to read each other's responses and be able to reply to students from other schools regarding the cases, thus teaching each other how to see the cases from differing perspectives.

Cases include a wide range of issues, from communication issues such as how to break bad news and admit mistakes, to dealing with "noncompliant" patients and patients seeking to integrate complementary and alternative medicine into their treatment plans, to responding with cultural sensitivity and competency to a diverse patient population or health care team. Cases have been written to provoke discussion of how a professional might word differences of opinion to encourage thoughtful, productive feedback rather than confrontation. Medical students will be reading and responding to comments on the cases by students from other schools, including nursing and public health. We will pair students at similar stages of training, for example, having third-year medical students discussing clinical vignettes with master's nursing students preparing to be nurse practitioners.

Finding the best way to teach ethics to clinical students has been the philosopher's stone for medical education. While many techniques have been tried with frustrating results, this is the first one to be embedded into the world of team-based clinical practice. Third-year clerkship students who are taught ethics alongside residents and nurses will be much more attentive and better able to internalize its lessons when they see its essential role in patient care.

Any ethics education in the first two years of medical school must be seen to be preparatory to later stages, and incomplete without follow-up in the clinical years. Ethics in the first two years might also be taught interprofessionally, either online or with an occasional small group activity that brings together nursing and medical students. But ethics must be taught in the third year, while students are immersed in clinical rotations, in order for the students to fully appreciate its relevance. Much the same can be said for all of the health care professions: trainees must be taught ethics (or ethics lessons must be reinforced) in the practice settings where they will spend their career, in order for the subject not to appear to be merely classroom learning—necessary for the test, but not for life (much like the Krebs cycle).

Teaching ethics well is absolutely essential in medical education, since seven out of the fourteen content directives from the LCME relate to ethics and professionalism. They specifically mention ethical principles, ethics of research, and societal problems such as violence and abuse, cultural insensitivity, and gender bias. And, importantly, each of the seven is a "must," not just a "should," which is defined as "absolutely necessary for the achievement and maintenance of accreditation."[4] These content directives are also important as they naturally prepare students for the development of four of the six ACGME core competencies, which also relate to ethics: patient care, interpersonal and communication skills, professionalism, and systems-based practice.

With the metaphor of the Bronze Age, we refer to the ancient myths of stages of history, wherein there is a historical progression, as well as anthropological observations of metallurgy. If we were to take the mythological metaphor too seriously, the analogy would break down most seriously in proposing that there was ever a Golden Age. Of course almost all grand accounts of human history are distorted by an imaginary idealized past. The Golden Age of bioethics, though, was a time when one person could master all the literature because it was so sparse, and use a single philosophical theory (or, sometimes, theology) to provide answers to all

---

[4]See Content Directives 10, 17, 19, 20, 21, 22, 23.

questions. Thanks to the enormous growth during the Silver Age, the field of healthcare ethics is much bigger now and much more complex.

The metaphor of the Bronze Age is meant to capture the sense that we now need to take stock of the complexity and discover (or recover) some themes that run through many subjects in order to prevent ethics from becoming so specialized that only experts or scholars feel at home with the subject. And while this approach is not revolutionary in the sense of proposing a new set of values or principles, interprofessional ethics may challenge the authority of people who have staked out a professionally defined territory; it is sufficiently challenging to the current profession-based paradigm that it deserves to be considered a new stage in ethics history. The future success of interprofessional ethics is by no means guaranteed—it will sometimes require a challenge within the academic bureaucracy (and some funding) to accomplish its goals.

The Bronze Age of bioethics is beginning to yield a new alloy of interprofessional ethics. We can and should be proud of this development. Yes, we should be grateful for the intellectual founders and builders of the field who inaugurated the Golden and Silver Ages, those who wrote the foundational texts of the field of bioethics and those who extended it into all of the health professions and medical specialties. Our task, even if more humble, is to discover and appreciate the value of working with more base metals like copper and tin to produce alloys, those who, in other words, have found ways to make the precious metals much more useful to human life, those who do the teaching, administration, and clinical work of the field each day but who are comparatively less recognized or appreciated. These practitioners and providers have laid the groundwork for a field that is becoming stronger and more malleable—and so with this book and our cases, we announce the inauguration of the Bronze Age of bioethics.

Acknowledgments Nathan Carlin from the McGovern Center at UTH was especially helpful in the drafting of this chapter, and deserves special acknowledgment as a co-author for his contributions to this chapter.

Suggestions for Further Reading

Brajtman, S., D. Wright, P. Hall, S.H. Bush, and E. Bekele. 2012. Toward better care of delirious patients at the end of life: A pilot study of an interprofessional educational intervention. *Journal of Interprofessional Care* 26(5): 422–425.

Deneckere, S., M. Euwema, C. Lodewijckx, M. Panella, T. Mutsvari, W. Sermeus, and K. Vanhaecht. 2013. Better interprofessional teamwork, higher level of organized care, and lower risk of burnout in acute health care teams using care pathways: A cluster randomized controlled trial. *Medical Care* 51(1): 99–107.

Freeth, D., and Interprofessional Education. 2007. *Association for the study of medical education*. Scotland, UK: Edinburgh.

Hoffman, S.J., and D. Harnish. 2007. The merit of mandatory interprofessional education for pre-health professional students. *Medical Teacher* 29(8): e235–e242.

Owen, J., T. Brashers, C. Peterson, L. Blackhall, and J. Erickson. 2012. Collaborative care best practice models: A new educational paradigm for developing interprofessional educational (IPE) experiences. *Journal of Interprofessional Care* 26(2): 153–155.

Pronovost, P., S. Berenholtz, T. Dorman, P.A. Lipsett, T. Simmonds, and C. Haraden. 2003. Improving communication in the ICU using daily goals. *Journal of Critical Care* 18(2): 71–75.

Shaw, S.N. 2008. More than one dollop of cortex: Patients' experiences of interprofessional care at an urban family health centre. *Journal of Interprofessional Care* 22(3): 229–237.

Stone, N. 2006. Evaluating interprofessional education: the tautological need for interdisciplinary approaches. *Journal of Interprofessional Care* 20(3): 260–275.

Yarborough, M., T. Jones, T.A. Cyr, S. Phillips, and D. Stelzner. 2000. Interprofessional education in ethics at an academic health sciences center. *Academic Medicine* 75(8): 793–800.

Chapter 2
Framing Interprofessional Ethics Cases

Introduction

Casebooks have long been a staple in programs of professional education that place a high value on the development of critical thinking and clinical judgment in practical decision making. They appear in curricula in a variety of forms, typically involving the common elements of a narrative: a brief description of context, several characters with complex motives, and a problem or obstacle that is open to multiple interpretations. The characters have assigned professional roles and expectations. The problems they face are intended to represent the normal range of challenges in professional life. And resolutions are judged by whether learned skills and principles have been applied appropriately and are consistent with the norms of sound practice.

This case method is well established in business, public administration, law, and throughout the health professions. Its strength, in socializing students to the ways of each particular profession, however, turns out to be its major weakness. Cases are written to apply to one profession at a time. Most are specialized in terminology and context. All invoke certain elements of a particular profession's point of view. Given that each student is entering only their own chosen profession, and the cases are written by a faculty member who belongs to that profession, the end result is almost too obvious to point out.

What has gone unnoticed until now, however, is that this makes the case method and casebooks irrelevant to the modern context of professional practice, where no one profession can assert complete control or confidence in mastery of all crucial features. Nowhere is this more apparent than in the health professions. Technology and increasing specialization have made health care into a team effort. The world of professional health care practice is increasingly an interprofessional place. Casebooks should follow suit.

Another development of note in professional education is the ascendency of responsible practice as a central theme. For some professions, this entails a code of

© The Author(s) 2016
J.P. Spike and R. Lunstroth, *A Casebook in Interprofessional Ethics*,
SpringerBriefs in Ethics, DOI 10.1007/978-3-319-23769-5_2

ethical conduct to be incorporated in everyday decision making. Ethics becomes a repository of tools and concepts that are useful in reading the signs of, and heading off, potential wrongdoing. In many of the health professions, the conduct of research has also been a prominent focus for ethics casebooks. Both case law and government regulations play large roles in setting expectations for biomedical research. Accordingly, much of the available case material supports efforts to ensure legal and regulatory compliance. Common to the other professions, these often organize case material by degree program. Again, the ethical issues faced by the interprofessional team receive no attention, despite the team's central role in professional practice: grant writing involves teams, as does the research conducted, and the authorship of the results. We intend to offer a casebook that focuses on problems at the intersection of professional practices, where teams and multiple codes of conduct meet.

Having multiple professions and their distinctive modes of practice represented in a single set of cases also adds the pragmatic advantage of versatility in adoption and use. As health curricula diversify to include a broader range of supporting specialties, cases with interprofessional issues are likely to be more relevant than those directed at a single profession. Including interprofessional cases is truer to today's practices, a recognition of the pluralism of perspectives across the professions. As each person learns ethics from our cases, he or she also learns about the other professions, their responsibilities, and their ethics. An interprofessional ethics, then, teaches a balanced representation of views.

Rather than assuming a single, underlying set of core principles from which all professions deduce their particular ethical variations, we embrace differences among the professions and assume that each adds a missing piece to a larger puzzle or enriches our understanding of the concepts represented by the core principles. There are clearly common elements to be found: some ethical claims and justifications shared across the professions and some facts that shape the contours of practice in shared domains. Still, there are advantages to apprehending the full range of ethical views across professions, especially in cases where mutual understanding is essential to any viable ethical resolution.

Interprofessionalism

With a commitment to pluralism, or at least to openness to the possibility of important contributions (either by adding principles or deepening our understanding of the potential meaning of principles) across professions, future or current health care professionals can avoid the mistake of treating any single ethical framework as sufficiently comprehensive to meet all of our needs. This commitment entails welcoming the opportunity to enter into discussions of normative ethics with members of other professions, to learn alternative approaches to justification for a choice of course of action, and to open each of the professions to new ideas and, potentially, new ways of thinking. We expect that this movement across each profession's ethical stands will have pedagogical value, exposing students to extramural ethical claims. More importantly, we believe that it is a necessary step in building a distinctive interprofessional approach to ethical issues.

The question is, what might an interprofessional approach to ethics look like? In simple terms, we can identify three ways to attempt to frame an answer. A consolidational frame would attempt to integrate or to bind separate professional views together into a unified whole, in some sense greater than the sum of its constituent parts. Interprofessional health care ethics, then, is understood as an amalgamation of medical, nursing, dental, and public health ethics, presumably with some safeguards for consistency. This type of unification serves as an antidote to the risk of conflicting values arising from the pluralism of health professions. Of course, it assumes a high degree of commensurability across professions.

A second frame is more essentialist than the logic of the consolidational view. It assumes that surface differences will give way to a small, shared set of basic principles held in common. This notion of an overlapping consensus has the effect of allowing us to reach a single core set that may or may not belong to any one of the given professions, but more closely resembles a unitary point of view. This strategy differs from the first as it would end up eventually converting ethical problems from interprofessional to intra-professional ones. While this may be desirable, it actually sidesteps the question of what an interprofessional ethics might look like by assuming there will only be one ultimate set of values for all professions.

A third frame, rather than falling between these two opposites, suggests a change in analytical focus. Attention shifts away from viewing the professions from an external vantage point in order to consolidate into a larger mixture, or to condense or reduce to an essence. In the third frame, interprofessional ethics emerges from the efforts of professionals to work out conciliatory resolutions in the face of disagreements and conflict. The tools and skills needed to affect these resolutions may characterize a distinctly interprofessional approach to ethical judgment that begins with accepting pluralism but then focuses on finding grounds (or a process) for collective agreement.

We do not choose from these three interpretations of interprofessional ethics. We offer tools that would allow any of them to blossom, beginning with general ethical *theories* that purport to be universally applicable (more like the second frame) and then present ethical *principles* that are more amenable to a pluralistic understanding of interprofessional ethics (more like the first frame). If, in the dialogue these tools foster, professions realize there are important ethical lessons they ought to adopt from other professions, that their own internal ethics were deficient, then perhaps the third frame will have been empirically vindicated.

No matter which frame seems most accurate, the ethical benefit comes from having students practice modes of judgment that prepare them to reason in deeper ways about bridging the divides that separate the ethical views of the professions. There should be room within the structure of different cases to invite a range of resolutions and to have these resolutions vary somewhat with the mix of students involved.

Different Levels of Ethical Issues in the Cases

Some simple cases are straightforward, where the emphasis is on basic recognition of relevant ethical features and concerns. Others cases are more complex, involving instances of genuine dilemmas, showing two different ethical features in tension. Both of these types of cases can be components of the cases we offer. However, our cases also present potential conflict among the ethical stands of two or more professions. We comment on each of these three levels of complexity in turn.

The straightforward elements in some cases are typically instances where self-interest is impinging on professional responsibility, or there may be some inadequate knowledge base (or self-deception), with excuses offered for avoiding an ethical responsibility. Drawing on a central existentialist term, these might be called cases of bad faith. The student is expected to uncover these in a diagnostic way and point to an appropriate course of action and rationale for it.

Some cases add complexity by bringing conflicting duties or competing values into play. Some will introduce the problem of scale, where conflicts range across levels of responsibility—from the client, to the organization, to the state, for example. These cases represent ethical dilemmas. Students then will be expected to analyze these situations, breaking them down into the components in conflict and justifying an ethical course of action.

The most complex cases build on the skills from the two earlier levels but require a capacity to assume different ethical points of view and to test resolutions across these. Recognizing bad faith and being able to resolve dilemmas prepares the student to address less tractable conflicts between competing ethical traditions and rival approaches to ethical judgment.

Since our intent is to build students' capacity for ethical judgment, we begin with a heuristic framework that represents a starting point for the consideration of each case. Organized as a series of questions, the framework can accommodate a wide range of normative approaches without being dogmatic or prejudicial. The idea is to provide some guidance that opens the student to ethical thinking, without closing off alternative approaches and concepts.

A Framework to Help Formulate Ethical Judgments

The case situations presented here are intended to evoke ethical judgments of different kinds. Before a judgment can be made about what should be done, a few simple questions can clear away features of the situation that are ethically irrelevant and can help focus reflection on what should count. The first question is to help establish the basic parameters of ethical consideration.

1. What are the ethically relevant features of the situation?
   An answer will require a thoughtful assessment of *prior commitments*—those
   agreements that create duties and obligations typically tied to important relationships, including familial ones, professional roles, and group memberships.
   A special class of obligations arises from *rights* that are typically assigned priority
   over other commitments. Are there any rights claims being made, or can you
   identify any? Or is there a common good or greater good that can be identified? This
   first question is a test of your ability to see the situation from all points of view.
   The next question gets to the core issue of ethical claims and regard for others. It
   is a test of your ethical sensitivity and imagination. To adequately answer these
   questions, one must be able to use your imagination to develop empathy,
   kindness, compassion.

2. What is at stake for all of those involved and for those who might be affected?
   This question requires an impartial stance so that our own personal interests do
   not get in the way of making a sound ethical judgment. You must put aside your
   own potential gains and losses in favor of a sensitive rendering of the possible
   effects on others—not just the others named in the situation but all others who
   might be affected by the action taken or avoided. This is known as the *ethical
   point of view*; it requires empathy to fully understand and appreciate the interests
   of others, especially of the socially and economically vulnerable, who are often
   overlooked. Now that you have identified the ethical nature of the problem with
   these first two questions, it is time to clarify the situation.
   There are limitations that can prevent you from being able to choose to act
   ethically.

3. Are there limits to the ethical responsibilities of those in the situation?
   Is there a single best action or stance that can be freely chosen? Or are the
   available choices constrained by external factors or an inability to see beyond
   one's own interest? Is the situation itself a product of unjust procedures or rules
   that fail to treat people with equal concern and respect? Is coercion present? This
   step is a test of your analytical and problem-solving skills, higher-level skills
   more like critical thinking than like factual knowledge retrieval. It tests the
   ability to recognize, confront and resolve subtle background assumptions that
   can obscure the ethical issues.
   At this point, you have made some judgment about what should be done. One
   last test is in order.

4. If the chosen action were to be generally observed, would the consequences and
   possible side effects still be reasonably acceptable to all those affected?
   This is a final test to ensure that the stakes mentioned in question 3 have been
   weighed from an ethical point of view. It ensures that the fairness of actions to
   others is given a central role in ethical judgment. This helps focus on your sense
   of obligations and responsibilities towards others, your personal attitude and
   willingness to assume responsibility and take some leadership. Test 4 is a check
   of your integrity, professionalism, and character.

Finally, attention needs to be given to improving the prospects for ethical action generally by addressing the institutional context and its contribution to unfairness and unjustifiable unequal treatment.

5. What are the implications of this situation for the justness of the institutions involved?

Do commitments and roles or rules and procedures need to be changed to protect the welfare or capacities of others for future ethical action? This is sometimes called organizational ethics, wherein a case brings to our attention a systematic problem with our system, organization, or policies and procedures. If the system somehow inhibits your ability to do what is right, you must then consider addressing those problems, trying to improve the system without endangering your effectiveness to work within it.

Sometimes a professional can pass the first four tests but be stymied (or think they are stymied) by the place where he or she works. This can lead to moral distress, a topic on which there is a large literature, mostly from nursing. Nurses often feel that they do not have the power or authority to change something they consider dangerous to patients or otherwise unethical. However, professionals from any field can feel burnout and moral distress from feeling as if they are being overworked and that their opinions are not respected by the hospital or health care system that employs them. Increasingly, we see the same concerns about moral distress voiced by physicians, as health care systems become larger and more centrally controlled.

To really succeed in any job, you must learn when and how you can contribute to improving the system and how not to be demoralized by moral distress when you can't— a test of your resilience.

Acknowledgments Stephen Linder from the School of Public Health at UTH was especially helpful in the drafting of this chapter, and deserves special acknowledgment as a co-author for his contributions to this chapter.

Suggestions for Further Reading

American Society of Bioethics and Humanities. 2009. *ASBH task force on ethics and humanities in undergraduate medical programs.* Glenview, IL: Author.

Aveyard, H., S. Edwards, and S. West. 2005. Core topics of health care ethics. The identification of core topics for interprofessional education. *Journal of Interprofessonal Care* 19(1): 63–69.

Berk, N.W. 2001. Teaching ethics in dental schools: Trends, techniques, and targets. *Journal of Dental Education* 65(8): 744–750.

Bertolami, C.N. 2004. Why our ethics curricula don't work. *Journal of Dental Education* 68(4): 414–425.

Burston, A.S., and A.G. Tuckett. 2012. Moral distress in nursing: Contributing factors, outcomes and interventions. *Nursing Ethics* 20(3): 312–324.

Caldicott, C.V., and E.A. Braun. 2009. Should professional ethics education incorporate single-professional or interprofessional learning? *Advances in Health Science Education* 16: 143–146.

Childs Jr, J.M. 1987. Interprofessional approach to ethical issues. *Theory into Practice* 26(2): 124–128.

Clark, P.G., Cott, C., and Drinka, T.J.K. 2007. Theory and practice in interprofessional ethics: A framework for understanding ethical issues in health care teams. *Journal of Interprofessional Care,* 21(6): 591–603.

Curran, V.R., D.R. Deacon, and L. Fleet. 2005. Academic administrators' attitudes towards interprofessional education in Canadian schools of health professional education [Supplemental material]. *Journal of Interprofessional Care* 19(s1): 76–86.

Ewashen, C., G. McInnis-Perry, and N. Murphy. 2013. Interprofessional collaboration-in-practice: The contested place of ethics. *Nursing Ethics* 20(3): 325–335.

Figley, C., Huggard, P., and Rees, C.E. 2013. *First do no self-harm*. Oxford: Oxford U Press.

Gardner, S.F., G.D. Chamberlin, D.E. Heestand, and C.D. Stowe. 2002. Interdisciplinary didactic instruction at academic health centers in the United States: Attitudes and barriers. *Advances in Health Sciences Education* 7: 179–190.

Gisondi, M.A., R. Smith-Coggins, P.M. Harter, R.C. Soltysik, and P.R. Yarnold. 2004. Assessment of resident professionalism using high-fidelity simulation of ethical dilemmas. *Academic Emergency Medicine* 11(9): 931–937.

Goelen, G., G. De Clercq, L. Huyghens, and E. Kerckhofs. 2006. Measuring the effect of interprofessional problem-based learning on the attitudes of undergraduate health care students. *Medical Education* 40: 555–561.

Irvine, R., I. Kerridge, J. McPhee, and S. Freeman. 2002. Interprofessionalism and ethics: Consensus or clash of cultures? *Journal of Interprofessional Care* 16(3): 199–210.

Jauhar, S. 2014. *Doctored*. New York: Farrar, Straus and Giroux.

Jennings, B. 2003. Introduction: A strategy for discussing ethical issues in public health. In *Ethics and Public Health: Model Curriculum*, ed. B. Jennings, J. Kahn, A. Mastroianni, and L.S. Parker, 1–12. Washington, DC: Association of Schools of Public Health.

Marcus, M.T., W.C. Taylor, M.D. Hormann, T. Walker, and D. Carroll. 2011. Linking service-learning with community-based participatory research: An interprofessional course for health professional students. *Nursing Outlook* 59: 47–54.

Poirier, T.I., and Wilhelm, M. 2013. Interprofessional education: Fad or imperative. *American Journal of Pharmaceutical Education* 77(4), Article 68.

Rafter, M.E., I.J. Pesun, M. Herren, J.C. Linfante, M. Mina, C.D. Wu, and J.P. Casada. 2006. A preliminary survey of interprofessional education. *Journal of Dental Education* 70(4): 417–427.

Sharp, H.M., R.A. Kuthy, and K.E. Heller. 2005. Ethical dilemmas reported by fourth-year dental students. *Journal of Dental Education* 69(10): 1116–1121.

Stoddard, H.A., and T. Schonfeld. 2011. A comparison of student performance between two instructional delivery methods for a health care ethics course. *Cambridge Quarterly of Health care Ethics* 20: 493–501.

Vanlaere, L., and C. Gastmans. 2007. Ethics in nursing education: Learning to reflect on care practices. *Nursing Ethics* 14(6): 758–766.

Vidette Todaro-Francheschi. 2013. *Compassion Fatigue and Burnout in Nursing*. NY: Springer.

Whitehead, C. 2007. The doctor dilemma in interprofessional education and care: How and why will physicians collaborate? *Medical Education* 41: 1010–1016.

Yarborough, M., T. Jones, T.A. Cyr, S. Phillips, and D. Stelzner. 2000. Interprofessional education in ethics at an academic health sciences center. *Academic Medicine* 75(8): 793–800.

Chapter 3
Using Ethical Theories as a Tool for Understanding Cases

Introduction: What Ethics Is, What Ethics Isn't, and When It All Began

Ethics is not the same thing as morality. For one thing, morality is more of a matter of accepted social conventions or religious traditions, without the requirement of any rational, empirical, or scientific justification. In fact, moral stances can appear somewhat arbitrary when they are unfamiliar within your culture. Furthermore, ethics is not the same thing as strongly held personal opinion, "gut feelings," the law, or compliance with regulations. Each of these may be confused with ethics, but none of them requires rational, empirical, or scientific justification, and each can be just as unethical as some of the social conventions called morality.

Ethics can be said to have begun at one particular place and time, when Socrates (469–399 BCE) asked a group in ancient Athens around 400 BCE, "Is something right because it is commanded by the Gods, or is it commanded by the Gods because it is right?" That simple question led to a quest to find a justification for morality beyond simply asserting that it is what the law says or what a priest says (which was much the same thing in those days).

Ethics, then, is the careful, reflective, critical and systematic study of values or "morality" whose goal is to identify *justified* ways of behaving and acting towards others. In the academic world, ethics is usually considered a branch of philosophy, which pursues the systematic study or search for the rational and empirical justifications of many different subjects (e.g., the philosophy of science, the philosophy of mathematics, the philosophy of psychology). Ethics, then, is the systematic study or search for rational and empirical justifications of how one should (ought to) treat other people or, more generally, how one should lead one's life. In other words, one might say ethics is the application of critical thinking skills and scientific evaluation of moral claims. Or, borrowing from popular medical pedagogy, one might say ethics is EBM: evidence based morality.

© The Author(s) 2016
J.P. Spike and R. Lunstroth, *A Casebook in Interprofessional Ethics*,
SpringerBriefs in Ethics, DOI 10.1007/978-3-319-23769-5_3

Ethics changes over time. That is not a disqualification for its counting as careful or systematic. Rather, one ought to hope it changes, making progress, as do medicine and science. A simple, classic example of ethical progress involves the issue of slavery. While the unethical practice of slavery was widely accepted from Biblical times through the writing of the American Constitution, it is now recognized as a grave violation of human rights. Even today some people express doubts at a theoretical level about whether ethics can ever be universal; however, few people today would protest that the claim that slavery is wrong is culturally relative. There is a deep lesson there: do not allow the unquestionable fact that we are not perfect lead to cynicism or let it stop you from trying to improve yourself, your profession, or your society.

Some who doubt the universality of ethics bring what they think is historical sophistication to their argument by suggesting that Western ideas dominate bioethics. There is much truth to that claim. Modern science also originated in Europe, with Newton and Boyle in the late 1600s, through the 1800s with Dalton, Darwin, and Mendeleev. But that is not a valid argument against the validity of either science or ethics. The geographical origin of such theories alone cannot invalidate their claims—they had to come from somewhere. (Indeed, the claim that the historical origin of a theory invalidates it is known in logic as "the naturalistic fallacy.") The important thing is that important science is now done everywhere, using the same methodology, and we ought to expect the same from ethics.

Additionally, the Enlightenment was not just a time of sudden, accidental realization or discovery of some unethical practices; it was a time when careful philosophical reflection on accepted practices led to important changes regarding which of those traditions were considered acceptable. With philosophers from John Locke and Bento (or Baruch) Spinoza in the late 1600s, through David Hume and Immanuel Kant in the late 1700s, and into the late 1800s with John Stuart Mill, the human race awoke from a dogmatic slumber (to borrow a famous phrase from Kant).

In many ways, some people still struggle with the changes, finding it harder to overcome behaviors and beliefs that seem important socially (or just valuable personally) even if they are ethically unjustifiable. It could be that the longer one has behaved in a certain manner, the less willing one becomes to accept that it is wrong—a simple defense mechanism to preserve one's self-respect. But that too is no argument that a practice is ethically justified.

The better lesson for all people to accept would be that, because ethics changes over time, we must all accept a dose of humility. Entire civilizations and cultures have been blind to terrible injustices, and there is no guarantee that we are not still ignorant of others.

Indeed, one could better argue that Western countries (and the United States in particular) have become leaders in bioethics because they have been more willing to admit their mistakes, sometimes only after a lengthy investigation and news coverage. This is quite the opposite from believing themselves superior and imposing their views "imperialistically" on others; leadership in ethics is more closely related to publically admitting past failures and proposing ways to reduce the likelihood that such events will be repeated in the future. Others who follow the lessons we offer are then best understood as demonstrating the wisdom of learning from our mistakes, rather than self-righteously denying that they are susceptible to the same biases that led to our own ethical errors.

Still, it must be admitted that a universal ethical consensus is rare. For the most part, there is often a strong consensus among professionals in the countries of England, the United States, Canada, and Australia. A common culture and a common language no doubt contribute to making it easier to arrive at that consensus. If that was all there was to it, it would not suffice for that consensus to count as an ethical consensus.

However, that is not all there is to it: depending somewhat on the topic discussed, the ethical consensus typically represents not just the United States and other English-speaking nations but also of many European professional societies and the World Health Organization. In addition, developed countries in Asia, the Middle East, and the Southern Hemisphere have shown increasing interest in and willingness to adopt similar ethical principles and the conclusions they generate— the world is (in other words) increasingly recognizing that ethical principles have a strong claim to universal applicability and validity, regardless of their historical or geographical origins.[1]

Ethical Theories

It is natural to hope to discover a single, simple ethical theory that would enable us to answer every ethics question definitively. Unfortunately, no such theory exists, and most likely never will.

A number of great philosophers of the past proposed such ethical theories. Many of their theories still survive, though each theory has evolved over time. There are ethics textbooks that will lead you through many of these theories, but that is not the goal of this book. Our goal is not so much to understand complex philosophical theories, and the arguments in support of each of them, but to focus on improving our skills at solving current ethical conundrums and dilemmas.

To seek one theory, or one system, that will answer all of our ethical questions, so that we can input data and output answers like a science, would be naïve at any rate. Ethics is more of a human science or a field of the humanities. It cannot be precisely quantified, and its methodology combines logical argument, human experience, and semantics (careful analysis of the meaning of terminology) as much as measurement.

---

[1]See B. Baker and S. Latham, et al., ed. *The American Medical Ethics Revolution: How the AMA's Code of Ethics Has Transformed Physicians' Relationships to Patients, Professionals, and Society.* JHU Press, 1999.

In ethics, as in the natural and human sciences, it is very important to have a healthy skepticism; we must seek evidence for claims. For guidance we may consider all of the well-established ethical theories, but also draw from other practical sources of information, such as economics, public policy, psychology, sociology, and anthropology.

When we sense a convergence of evidence and arguments upon one conclusion we can publish our results. As the discussion involves more people, and differences narrow with a more refined understanding of the source of differences, a consensus is gradually reached. The validity of the arguments is being tested, as it were, as well as the consequences of various choices. After years of such reflection, a broad social agreement evolves. John Rawls, a very important twentieth century philosopher referred to this as "wide reflective equilibrium."

This approach may seem less than fully satisfying to some people. Many novices hope to be given a simple theory or logarithm (perhaps in an introductory chapter of a textbook like this) they can apply to all of their information about a case in the hope that with it they will be able to mechanically generate a single correct answer. However, there is no single, universally accepted theory. If there were, there would be little need to read and discuss cases in order to refine one's skills of reflection, analysis, and resolution regarding difficult situations.

In fact, there never will be such a theory since human nature and society are too complex to be fully captured by any single theory. Difficulty is also inevitable since we are discussing cases with multiple agents, where each agent has diverse and often conflicting interests. Instead of there being one right answer, often there are many competing reasonable answers, and what is needed is the experience and wisdom to decide which factors are most important.

The Two Modern Philosophical Theories of Ethics

The lack of a single triumphant theory of ethics is not to disparage philosophers. Ethics has benefited from their theories, and it could even be argued that there would be no ethics without philosophy. Philosophy is the intellectual effort to clarify and justify claims in a way that must be acceptable to everyone without any cultural, religious, or political presuppositions. There have been two seminal philosophical ethical theories engaged in a debate over the past 150 years; each has further evolved by learning from the challenges posed by the other theory.

These two theories, worth an entire semester-long college course, are called Utilitarianism and Deontology. They are each one-sided in ways that the other theory helps to complete. But there is no way to combine the two; they are, as philosophers like to say, incommensurable. More colloquially, they are like oil and water: they cannot be mixed together in order to form a simple solution. Thus the theories and their differences are worth a quick synopsis.

Each of these two modern theories has a seminal theorist. For **Deontology**, it is Immanuel Kant. Kant's ethics privileges rationality and formulates "the moral law" in the terms of universal maxims, or guiding principles we would expect everyone to agree to if they were rational. Kant hoped to defend many Christian values by demonstrating that they were rational rather than revealed. A paraphrase of his ultimate rule, the Categorical Imperative, is "Respect others' goals in life, and never treat them merely as a means to your own ends," or (he thought this amounted to the same thing) "Only act according to rules which you would be willing to require everyone else in the world to follow."[2]

For **Utilitarianism**, ethics is defined by choosing actions that maximize pleasure and happiness and minimize pain and suffering. Its most famous proponent is John Stuart Mill who summarized the central principle of Utilitarianism as doing "the greatest good for the greatest number of people." Utilitarianism regards ethics as an empirical or scientific subject, and a natural part of policy debates. For example, "how many people would be affected by a change in public policy?" and "how much would it help them?" are the sorts of questions Utilitarians think are essential to deciding the most ethical course of action. Beginning over 150 years ago in England, Utilitarians fought against child labor and slavery, and in favor of free public schools, universal health care, women's right to vote, and animal welfare (the latter because, from the beginning, pain and suffering in all sentient beings counted, and hence included animals as well as people as legitimate objects of ethical concern).

The easiest way to understand the difference between these two theories is to examine how they approach ethical arguments and justifications. Deontology is a theory of *a priori* truths, eternal, unchanging and universal—in the same intellectual category of knowledge as mathematics and logic. In contrast, Utilitarianism judges an action by its consequences, and so its conclusions are *a posteriori*, require empirical justifications, and are by definition context sensitive. Despite their differences, or perhaps *because* of them, both theories are vital for understanding ethics (and neither could replace the other).

Because of the fundamentally different nature of their arguments and justification, it would be impossible to construct a single theory that combines these two ethical theories. But most of us can draw help from both theories. And fortunately, both theories agree on the best or right thing to do in almost all cases. The truth is, it is only the unrelenting (or relentless) dedication of philosophers arguing for one theory over all others that has produced wonderful test cases to demonstrate where the two theories would diverge in their recommendations. Those test cases, such as the trolley problem, are well worth looking up online (and are covered in every

---

[2]Many people notice how much this sounds like the so-called Golden Rule in Christianity, "do unto others as you would have them do unto you." But it is equally similar to other, even more ancient religious texts such as the Hebrew Torah, Confucius' Analects, and the Mahabharata—all from around 600–900 BCE. So it may well be that all religious traditions support the claim of Kant that this is the most fundamental rule of ethics.

philosophy department ethics course). But since we are not out to choose between the two theories, we do not need to review them here.[3]

Practical ethics might best conclude neither utilitarianism nor deontology can be considered complete, and consider that they are each necessary, and jointly sufficient. Various ethicists react differently to the lack of a grand unifying theory of ethics. But intellectually it is no more problematic than the lack of a grand unified theory in physics. There is no reason to become disillusioned with the whole idea of ethical theory, or to feel compelled to choose one to put all of one's faith in and then ridicule the other. Physics is a solid science, with many proven theories, and very useful, even though it is clearly incomplete, and might never achieve a unified theory.

That these two modern theories are still the most important can be seen by their contemporary followers and defenders. The most famous contemporary deontologist is John Rawls, while the most famous contemporary Utilitarian is Peter Singer. Both are very influential, and deservedly so.[4]

In conclusion, one must resist the temptation to become an ideologue that adopts a simple system for generating answers to very complex and difficult cases, or, worse, trying to create examples just to prove your theory. In the professional world, our concern is to use ethical theories to help us with cases, and not the other way around.

Four Less Rigorous 'Alternative' Ethical Theories

There are other, less developed, ethical theories that also have adherents among the philosophically trained. For example, Aristotle's **virtue theory** provides a psychological account of the character traits one needs in order to have good judgment, right down to advice on how to raise a child. Everyone has probably heard of his doctrine of the golden mean between two extremes—e.g., courage is good, a virtue, but not recklessness or cowardice. Ultimately, according to Aristotle, the right thing to do in a situation is whatever a wise, experienced, and perceptive person with good practical judgment (*phronesis*) would do in the same situation. Virtue theory is especially appealing to people who believe that good role models are the

---

[3]One might even speculate that the choice between these two theories is a false dichotomy, that is, one must consider both in order to be completely fair to an issue. But so far there is no grand theory that shows how to make them compatible; it might be the ethical equivalent of light as a wave and as a particle in physics. At least, using that analogy, there is no reason to think one or both theories must be wrong, and the entire field is useless. Both physics and ethics are very important.

[4]Rawls great lifework was *A Theory of Justice*, Harvard U Press, Cambridge Mass, 1971. For scholars of Rawls, it is also important to read his later works, *Justice as Fairness*. Harvard Press, Cambridge, 2001, and *Political Liberalism*. Columbia U Press, NY, 1993. For Singer one might start with his *Animal Liberation* that first came out in 1975, and has had many editions, or his *The Expanding Circle: Ethics, Evolution, and Moral Progress,* Princeton U Press, New York, 2011.

essence of good teaching. The most famous contemporary virtue theorist in medicine is the physician Edmund Pellegrino.[5]

Another unique aspect of Aristotle's theory is the emphasis on not just knowing the right thing to do, a cognitive ability, but the importance of having the sort of character that does it ("gets it done"). This is captured in the Greek word for virtue, *arete*, more than in the English word "virtue"—for the Greeks virtue did not have moralistic undertones, but instead had a connotation of strength and success—a person who sets lofty goals and achieves them. Courage and generosity replace Christian virtues such as humility, chastity, and poverty.

The proliferation of interest in "leadership" might be taken as a sort of revival of virtue theory, but with less explicit emphasis on the ethics one expects from a good leader. Unfortunately the modern world has demonstrated that many successful leaders can be unethical, even tyrannical, and can lead to social disasters. Thus virtue theory's greatest value today might be to remind us all that good leaders need to be good in both senses, at getting things done and at being ethical. Virtue ethics also resonates deeply with many people interested in the way mentoring is an effective (or perhaps essential) tool in teaching ethics, that is, that one needs a good role model (again, good in both senses) in order to learn how to be ethical.

Other ethicists want to revive the medieval approach to ethics known as **casuistry**; comparing each new case to well-known and influential cases from the past, known as paradigm cases. One works through a new scenario by comparing it to past cases, and identifying any similarities and differences. In logic this is known as analogical reasoning. Casuistry is also an excellent description of most legal reasoning, especially case law; and since legal cases are central to almost every discussion of clinical and research ethics, clearly casuistry has a role in explaining the reasoning process of ethics.

On legal reasoning:
Legal reasoning is a form of humanistic and philosophical reasoning. Laws are products of a social consensus, and so are intended to represent a collective wisdom, and cases also bring in the judgment of 'the people' by their use of juries. The field of bioethics includes approximately equal numbers of people from medicine, philosophy, and the law. Using a law or a case as part of your ethical reasoning is perfectly acceptable. However when ethics is at issue, the law does not have the final say. Laws can be unethical, and so can be evaluated ethically just like other social conventions. Also, it is worth noting that in many clinical settings there is free advice from risk managers. But that too isn't always ethical. Remember most risk managers are not lawyers, and those that are have a client they represent—the hospital, not the clinician or the patient.

---

[5]Pellegrino, E.D., 1994. The Virtues and Obligations of Professionals. In: Beauchamp T.L., LeRoy W. ed., *Contemporary Issues in Bioethics*. Belmont, CA: Wadsworth Pub, pp 51–57.

Pearl:

Taking legal advice from a doctor is like taking medical advice from a lawyer
—George Annas, professor of Health Law.

The best known contemporary philosopher associated with casuistry is Al Jonsen and his co-author, Stephen Toulmin.[6]

Virtue theory and casuistry are two theories that are *older* than Utilitarianism and Deontology, but have contemporary adherents, and are still valuable. There are also two ethical theories that are *newer* than Utilitarianism and Deontology: feminist ethics and narrative ethics. Feminist ethics and narrative ethics do not propose systematic methods for defining right and wrong. As such, one might even question whether they should be counted as ethical *theories*. But they do both offer valuable advice about how to collect evidence or data before beginning an ethical analysis, and about what should even count as an ethical problem.

Feminist ethics stresses the importance of seeing through economic interests and social power structures, as well as giving the interests of minorities, and the poor and disempowered their due. Sometimes this is expressed as an "ethics of caring," and treats emotions like empathy or compassion as the core human qualities that enable sound ethical decision-making. The first philosopher to make "sympathy" for the suffering for others the foundation for philosophical ethics was David Hume, in the 18th century—before Kant or Mill.[7]

Dr. John Gregory wrote a book "Lectures Upon the Duties and Qualifications of a Physician," that many consider the first book of modern medical ethics, and first appeared in 1772. Many of these ideas also carried over into the book that coined the phrase 'medical ethics,' written soon after in 1791 by Dr. John Percival at the request of a hospital, and published in 1803 with the title "Medical Ethics: A Code of Precepts for the conduct of Physicians and Surgeons." Gregory and Percival agreed doctors ought to treat patients with sympathy, honesty (never deceit), respect, and see them as their equals and be their advocates. They repeatedly stressed the importance of a doctor having "empathy" or a "tender bond" to their patients.

Hume and his medical descendants can be considered the progenitors of what has come to be called an ethics of care, which has more recently come to be considered the earliest feminist theory of ethics. In contrast, some of the other books often considered the first works of feminist ethics, such as Mary Wollstonecraft's *Vindication of the Rights of Women* (1792) and John Stuart Mill

---

[6]*The Abuse of Casuistry*, Albert Jonsen and Stephen Toulmin, U California Press, Berkeley, 1988.
[7]*A Treatise of Human Nature*, 1739 and his *An Enquiry Concerning the Principles of Morals*, 1751. Hume's ethics are sometimes skipped over in philosophy department ethics courses because of the need to cover Kant and Mill, who both came soon after Hume (and were both influenced by him). But in medical ethics, that would be a mistake because of Hume's close friend, the physician John Gregory. Hume was also the most important philosopher in what is called 'the Scottish Enlightenment' (which came before, and very much influenced the Enlightenment in France).

and Harriet Taylor's *On the Subjection of Women* (1869) appeared after Hume, and so might be considered a natural development of ideas that were 'in the air' in Scotland and England. However these later books frame issues explicitly with regards to the rights of women in society, and so deserve the label of feminist while Hume and Gregory represent philosophical precursors with a more universal or medical focus.

For Hume, the essential point was much like contemporary evolutionary psychology, that we have a natural sympathetic reaction when we see someone suffering, and we all benefit from that being a human instinct. Hence ethics is natural and has a biological and emotional basis, and being ethical does not require great effort to overcome a normal state of egocentrism or selfishness.[8]

Nursing ethics, when presented as essentially different from medical ethics, was once taken to be an "ethics of care." The core claim was that both deontology and utilitarianism were coldly logical, and ignored the natural and emotional basis of 'moral sentiments.' Some authors interpreted "care" and "caring" as a quality that is a natural strength of women more than men, perhaps related to their maternal roles.[9,10]

Contemporary feminist ethics is more likely to replace the ethics of care with an ethics of redress of power to members of vulnerable groups including, but not limited to, women. And the nursing ethics literature has followed a similar path, with far less emphasis on a special ethics of care and more on the importance of patient advocacy.[11]

Narrative ethics is a very recent addition to the ethics literature. It stresses the importance of understanding people's choices as a function of a lifetime of events, circumstances, and decisions that make a person who s/he is today. Its advice is to better understand the individual person before applying any ethical generalizations; this pertains to the doctor, nurse, or dentist as well as the patient. One ought to know oneself and one's patient's personal history before making any recommendations. The primary proponents of this approach have come from the medical humanities, especially literature and medicine. They use the language of cultural anthropology to bolster their claim that we are all the products of cultural influences

---

[8]For interesting contemporary views of the idea that ethics is natural, and emotional, see J.D. Trout, *Why Empathy Matters: The Science and Psychology of Better Judgment* (Penguin Books, New York, 2010), the interdisciplinary research in *Moving Beyond Self-Interest* by S.L. Brown, M. Brown, and L.A. Penner (Oxford, 2012), and the entertaining narrative *The Empathy Exams* by Leslie Jamison (Graywolf Press, Minneapolis, 2014).

[9]Carol Gilligan's book *In a Different Voice*, Harvard UP 1993, set off much discussion about ethics as a part of psychological development, as she critiqued earlier work on the subject by Kohlberg as inherently sexist. However other feminist authors protested that this claimed 'strength' was a double-edged sword, implying that it opens the door to the insulting claim that women are by nature less 'rational' than men, and to the self-contradiction/absurdity/paradox of nurses being "ordered to care."

[10]SM Reverby, *Ordered to Care: The Dilemma of American Nursing, 1850–1945,* Cambridge U Press, Cambridge England, 1987.

[11]Laura Purdy, *Reproducing Persons*, Ithaca NY, Cornell Press, 1996.

(for better or, often, for worse) which must be identified and dealt with if decisions are to be made fairly.[12]

To compare these two most recent additions to the ethical literature, contemporary feminist ethics tends to focus on external (e.g. socio-economic) forces whereas narrative ethics focuses more on internal (e.g. personal, psychological) forces that help you understand a situation more deeply than a quick assessment or statement of "just the facts."[13]

Both narrative and feminist ethics can be taken as modern extensions of casuistry in advising that we understand cases from the ground up, being sensitive to the details that make one case different from another. But unlike casuistry, these modern (or 'postmodern') additions stress that we need to be critical of how the facts of a case are initially presented. One must be cautious and ask whether some perspectives or interpretations are being privileged over others, e.g., whether the power structure is being allowed to define what the problem is, while marginalizing the perspectives of other stakeholders. In the words of the populist movement of the 1960s, to be ethical one must be willing to sometimes "question authority" rather than presume its validity. How things first appear may be more a reflection of socio-economic differences than of justice.

None of these four alternative theories are wrong. But none of them could stand alone as a complete and universal ethical theory the way that Utilitarianism and Deontology claim. They are best seen as methodological supplements, since the two most philosophically powerful theories give so little guidance on how to apply them to real life. A good metaphor to explain their status: they are better treated like complementary medicine rather than alternative medicine, a supplement rather than a replacement for the more rigorously tested ethical theories.

Curiosity about all ethical theories is praiseworthy so long as it does not devolve into an ideological search for certainty in ethics. One may take an ethics course to learn more about any of these theories, but if any course makes one theory or another appear to be the sole or obvious preference, and treats others as if they were incoherent, the course (or instructor) is most likely biased. Each of the theories is interesting, reasonable, and valuable, but not exclusively so.

That there are two competing powerful theories of ethics, and (at least) four potentially valuable supplements, might make ethics seem rather uncertain and useless. But it isn't. It is better to have a few different ways to step out of your subjective opinions and more objectively analyze a conflict and develop a resolution than to have none at all and choose to 'trust your gut feelings.'

However for the fields of applied ethics in health care, especially the two major fields of clinical ethics and research ethics, you never are required to use theories for cases. Since a simpler system is available, it is easy to appreciate why it has

---

[12]Clifford Geertz's 1973 book *The Interpretation of Cultures,* New York: Basic Books, was an important influence, identifying the need for "thick descriptions" to understand human behavior.

[13]For more on narrative ethics, see Howard Brody, *Stories of Sickness,* second edition (2003), Oxford U Press, or Rita Charon and Martha Montello, ed., *Stories Matter: The Role of Narrative in Medical Ethics,* Routledge (New York, 2002).

been widely adopted. That's why the principles introduced in the next chapter are so popular. That doesn't mean you can't use ethical theories if you wish. They can help us understand what is at stake, ethically. But for most people faced with an ethical problem or a true dilemma, the principles will be the natural starting point.

Chapter 4
Using Principles as a Tool
for Understanding Ethics Cases

The Original Four Principles

For clinical ethics, the model used most often, even if it is less a theory than a
practical compromise, is called "the four principles." Tom Beauchamp and James
Childress first popularized this approach in their 1979 book, *Principles of
Biomedical Ethics*. They have continued to develop this account for nearly 40 years
and six editions. The principles have great utility, as evidenced by how they have
been adopted (with varying degrees of modifications) by textbooks in medical
ethics, nursing ethics, dental ethics, dental hygiene ethics, and many other clinical
fields. Indeed, there is no reason to think they should not apply equally well to all
clinical fields, and so could be useful for clinical social work and clinical psychology, as well as pharmacy, physical therapy, occupational therapy, speech
therapy, and other allied health professions. This also means they are especially
useful for helping an interprofessional team reach a consensus. Given the proven
utility of the approach for clinical ethics and research ethics, four additional principles are proposed to define professionalism, followed by four additional principles
for Public Health ethics.

"It's the principle of the thing" and "he's a man of principle" are examples of
how we naturally use the concept of principles in our everyday discourse about
ethics, more than we refer to any ethical theory.

What we have seen over nearly 40 years is that using the four Principles is
sufficient and satisfactory for most people. That is not to say any approach,
including the principles, will get everything right, but the failures usually have more
to do with internal resistance to change from individuals ('that's not how we were
taught in the good old days') or systems (that's not the financially most efficient, or
doesn't follow a policy already in place). In other words, to make the ethical
analysis more complex will not usually help make the people or institutions
involved more ethical. What is more important is to practice admitting issues in our
lives and work as ethical in nature, and become more sensitive at addressing those

© The Author(s) 2016
J.P. Spike and R. Lunstroth, *A Casebook in Interprofessional Ethics*,
SpringerBriefs in Ethics, DOI 10.1007/978-3-319-23769-5_4

issues ethically. For the truth is that many people wish to avoid conflicts, and this makes them hesitant to identify conflicts as ethical. For example, people will sometimes say a problem is "just" a problem with communication, because that avoids having a serious discussion about one's own values and goals and how they may conflict with those of other people.

The four principles in Beauchamp and Childress are respect for autonomy, beneficence, non-maleficence, and justice. Each principle can be justified by both of the ethical theories of deontology and utilitarianism, and hence have a strong claim to universality or universal acceptability.

Beauchamp and Childress describe their four principles as "mid-level principles," meaning each is less abstract than a theory, and makes no claim to being sufficient as a stand-alone principle. Thus it is always an error when someone says of a case that it is "an Autonomy case" as if only one principle is relevant. The principles have been widely adopted in hundreds of articles and textbooks, representing all healthcare professions. Recognizing the relevance of all four principles also reminds us that an important strength of this approach is that the principles of beneficence and non-maleficence represent the traditional values of medicine, or what some might think of as Hippocratic ethics, while the other two principles, autonomy and justice, represent more modern ethical values.[1]

The principles have also been simplified into a formula known as "the four boxes," which does not differ greatly in substance, but is a more appealing approach for some clinicians. While the four principles are more of an explanatory model, the four boxes appear to describe how to operationalize the four principles.[2]

Here is a brief summary of the four principles, with some elaborations by the editor of this book. Each can be understood as including both an aspirational ethical ideal and (*at least*) a minimal ethical (or sometimes, legal) duty.[3]

Autonomy: From the Greek, meaning self-determination. The clinician ought to provide all the relevant information to patients with decision-making capacity in order to empower patients to make an informed decision. The patient is the ultimate authority on what is best for his or her well-being because that is a value judgment; not everyone with the same illness would agree on the same treatment plan. While this does not mean patients can make any request, *at the very least*, though, it means patients with capacity have the *right to refuse* any recommendation.

---

[1] Some commentators refer to the four principles approach as "principlism," but the term originated with detractors of the approach (rather in the way opponents to the Affordable Care Act have called it "Obamacare") so this text refrains from using that term.

[2] See: A.R. Jonsen, M. Siegler, and W.J. Winslade (2002) *Clinical Ethics: A Practical Approach to Ethical Decisions in Clinical Medicine*, 4th Edition. New York: McGraw-Hill, Inc.

[3] These are the principles identified by Beauchamp and Childress in their book *Principles of Biomedical Ethics*. I do not quote the original source verbatim, but provide my own interpretations and elaborations. It is my addition to elaborate each principle as including both a positive ideal to aspire to and a minimal responsibility one must meet. Cf. T.L. Beauchamp and J.F. Childress (2009) *Principles of Biomedical Ethics*, Sixth Edition. New York: Oxford University Press. An interesting bit of trivia that might not be trivial: Beauchamp is a utilitarian and Childress is a deontologist. Each thinks that all four principles can be justified by both theories.

This principle changes the role of the clinician from being an authoritative expert to being an educator, which requires strong communication skills. Currently the preferred model of decision-making is called shared decision-making, though that does not mean the doctor has a 50–50 say in the answer; it means the doctor has an essential role in helping the patient understand his illness and all of the reasonable treatment options in order to help the patient make a decision that is best suited to the patient's goals of treatment. This is exactly what most patients want from their doctor.

The principle of autonomy only refers to patient autonomy, and is the natural result of recognizing patient's rights and the legal doctrine of informed consent. It is not about professional autonomy (which is addressed in the second set of four principles, with professional integrity). Autonomy also offers no direct guidance for decisions involving patients who lack capacity to make autonomous decisions. However one could charitably interpret it as counseling that clinicians should *at least* try to respect the less well informed or articulated preferences and behaviors of incapacitated persons into the treatment plan, and also that clinicians should try to find out from friends and family members of patients what the patient would want in cases where the patient cannot communicate. This is called substituted judgment.[4]

Some groups have protested that Autonomy has become the pre-eminent principle, trumping all the others. For example some have said that Asian cultures put the family's wishes before the patient's wishes. That is based largely on misunderstanding not just of the principle of Autonomy, but how the principles are supposed to work as a group. The importance of Autonomy comes from its role in allowing decisions to be individualized to the patient. So, in a pluralistic country with patients from many different cultures and religions, it is natural for Autonomy to be very important. What a Muslim patient and a Buddhist patient would choose in the same situation might be very different, and it is the principle of Autonomy that gives each of them the right to choose for themselves. Autonomy also gives a patient the right to say 'I want my family to do what they feel is best,' or to do what they feel obligated to do for reasons of filial piety. Autonomy is the principle that gives patients the right to choose to put the family's needs ahead of their own preferences.

In the U.S. and many other countries the legal doctrine of informed consent reinforces the import of Autonomy. A patient or a surrogate must agree to an intervention before it can be done. This too could be part of why Autonomy appears to some people to be more important than the other three principles. Informed consent requires (at the very least) that the decision maker know the chances of success of any recommended intervention, and all of the reasonable alternatives, before any consent can be considered informed.

---

[4]The four boxes uses the term "Patient Preferences."

Has Autonomy gone too far?

Why is the Principle of Respect for Autonomy so important, and why do so many people seem to think it has become too important, dominating the other principles?

What Autonomy protects more than anything else is pluralism. For example, it gives adult Jehovah's Witnesses the right to refuse transfusions. But it isn't just Jehovah's Witnesses, it gives us all a say in our own medical care to the degree we want to participate in the decision-making process and are capable of doing so.

So who would dislike that? There are a few reasons some people have suggested Autonomy has gone too far, and if we look at each one we will see we should give them far less credence than we typically do. Adding Autonomy to the more traditional principles brought medical ethics into the modern world.

1. *Religious absolutists might hate autonomy as it denies them the right to insist their views are true for everyone. Thus if Jehovah's Witnesses ruled the world, denying autonomy would mean no one could get blood transfusions, and if some sects of ultra-Orthodox Islam or ultra-Orthodox Judaism ruled the world then no one could ever be an organ donor or the recipient of an organ transplant. I don't think many people want such a world, or think it would be more ethical, though we want to respect the wishes of those who have those beliefs. Such respect for different beliefs is just what Autonomy encourages.*

2. *Some ultra-rationalist ethicists might also resent respecting Autonomy, as it gives too much respect to irrational beliefs, cultural artifacts such as the arbitrary religious traditions imposed on children by their parents at a young age. Autonomy encourages respect for such beliefs, on the assumption that people have the right to determine what happens to their own body in the medical system, rather than relying only on the (hopefully well-supported) scientific beliefs of doctors. It is hoped that by the time a person has reached adulthood they have had the ability to review their beliefs and choose which to follow.*

3. *People from very homogeneous societies might not see why we must respect the beliefs of people who belong to minority groups. But every country has at least a few minority groups, and it is only a question of whether they are recognized and respected. Autonomy protects the rights of members of each of those groups.*

4. *Lastly, there is the widespread claim that many Asian cultures, and Hispanic cultures, and other groups believe more in the family as decision maker than the individual. But Autonomy is also the best ethical defense for these groups: for it gives each individual the right to choose someone else to make their medical decisions, whether their spouse, their oldest son, their daughter in law, or a religious leader. All of these choices are*

deserving of respect by virtue of its being the choice of the patient. (Would we really want it any other way, i.e. where we let the family choose without first consulting the patient? What if the patient has always felt oppressed?) The right to have a member of your family make decisions is like the right to have your religious leaders decide: it is defended by the Principle of Autonomy, and so a reason to preserve that principle. Hence even believers in traditional value systems should be cautious before joining often careless and superficial criticisms of Autonomy.

Beneficence: The clinician ought to do what is medically determined to be in the patient's best interest, balancing the benefits and burdens of each treatment option for the patient. This is an altruistic principle, as it rules out any clinician letting one's own self-interest or third party interests (e.g., a hospital or an insurance company) interfere with what is best for the patient.

The principle of Beneficence identifies the clinician as a fiduciary, meaning that the clinician must always put the patient's best interest ahead of her own. If altruism seems to ask too much of the clinician by demanding that she be heroic (i.e., perform supererogatory acts), *at least* she must not allow vanity, fear of litigation, or her chosen specialty to bias her into underestimating the risks of an intervention for a patient.[5]

Non-maleficence ("Do No Harm"): The clinician must include preventing or relieving pain and/or other symptoms in the equation. Non-maleficence may counsel that hospice or palliative care is the best available treatment choice. Non-maleficence is a conservative principle meant to *at least* avoid taking unnecessary risks or performing heroic interventions that may make things worse, protracting someone's pain or suffering. It can also be interpreted to include a warning to know one's professional limits and to not attempt things that are beyond one's skills or training.[6]

Justice: Justice is the most complex and least intuitive of the four principles. It can be seen as both a positive duty requiring that we give vulnerable people the same care as powerful people (or, *at least*, try to reduce the health disparities between rich and poor), and as a negative duty requiring that we are careful stewards of our resources (or, *at least*, to make sure there is enough to take care of the minimal needs of everyone). These are sometimes identified as distributive justice, or the just distribution of a good like health care. Overall, at a minimum, justice tells us to take care of and to protect the vulnerable and least well off.[7]

---

[5]The four boxes uses the term "Best Interest."

[6]The four boxes use the term, "Quality of Life." That do no harm might be the most important of the principles can be explained by the fact that it is the only negative principle, something one ought not do, rather than what one ought to do. The Indian concept of *ahinsa* is a strong analogue, and central to much 'Eastern' ethics.

[7]The four boxes use the term "Contextual Features," a generic term that includes economic factors, religious factors, etc. This term in particular is so vague, a generic grab-bag, that I prefer the terminology of the four principles. In particular, justice is a very important ethical concept, as we

While defining the limits to justice may be difficult, it is important to acknowledge that it has ancient roots, and that doctors accepted a responsibility to care for the indigent throughout history (indeed, since Hippocrates). To turn away a patient for lack of ability to pay would be condemned in any epoch. And that altruism has been recognized in modern times by the AMA and built into the very definition of being a medical professional. A good discussion question can thus often be formed by asking if other professions ought to have similar responsibilities to the poor, mentally ill, or uninsured (to take three examples).[8,9]

From an interdisciplinary perspective, the members of a health care team might try to keep an overall balance by each advocating for one of the principles. Perhaps the doctor would choose to represent beneficence (the best interest of the patient from a medical point of view), the nurse might understand the role of patient advocate as requiring her to be vigilant about avoiding interventions with high risk or a low probability of success in the name of nonmaleficence, and justice might be the domain of the social worker who often considers financial issues as well as family dynamics and cultural context. Autonomy would be honored by including the patient as an equal partner in the team's decision-making process.

Even using this interdisciplinary team model, it is always important to remember that everyone on the team should be aware of the importance of all four principles. No case is "just" an autonomy case or "just" a nonmaleficence case. The only way to do a good job understanding a case is to carefully weigh how all four principles apply. Each of the four principles is considered to be relevant *prima facie*, which means that "on the face of it" each principle is part of any complete ethical analysis. It is also equally important to realize that they are four independent principles, which means they can conflict with each other. Thus, they are better thought of as helping you understand why some cases are complex than as a way of (over) simplifying cases.

(Footnote 7 continued)

will see in our elaboration of public health ethics. To replace "Justice" with "contextual features" is to hamstring the clarity of the ethical enterprise. For a sample of how the concept of justice has been the central philosophical concept in philosophical ethics, see the preeminent work of the twentieth century in the field: *A Theory of Justice*, by John Rawls (Harvard U Press, 1971). For a sample of how justice applies to health care, one can start with the collection *Medicine and Social Justice*, 2e. R Rhodes, MP Battin, and A Silvers, edd. Oxford UP, Oxford, 2012).

[8]See, for example, "Caring for the Poor," AMA Council for Ethical and Judicial Affairs, *JAMA*, 1993; 269:19; 2533–2537.

[9]The limit that no one can define is how altruistic one needs to be. Duties to the poor are commonly part of the definition of a profession, but getting paid enough to make a living is also part of the definition, so one cannot be expected to donate all of one's time to people who can't pay. The minimum ethical responsibility might devolve into support for improvements in the system so there are fewer people who require charity. Doctors mostly acknowledge this duty, but as an ethical principle it should apply equally to all health care professionals. If a doctor expresses any doubts, one might point out that the best law firms require at least 10 % of time be *pro bono*. And everyone in the health care field likes to think they are more ethical than lawyers!

A clinical ethics pearl:
If you are thorough, almost every ethics case will have some hidden surprises that will be discovered only after you get involved. That is why it is a mistake to try to resolve a case quickly. If you cut corners to resolve cases quickly (e.g., with just a phone call), it will be noticed by others (your teachers or, later, your patients). To do something ethically means taking no shortcuts. Rather than make it easier, it might make the task harder, but make the outcome more complete, fair and objective.

Lastly, a humorous mnemonic that may help you to remember the names of the four principles (autonomy, beneficence, nonmaleficence, and justice) is "Anywhere but New Jersey." It's silly, but it works!

On the ethics of research involving human subjects or participants:
The Belmont Report is the single most seminal document in research ethics concerning research on human subjects. Written at about the same time as The Principles of Biomedical Ethics, it proposed only three principles. For the purposes of this introduction, the most important fact to consider about The Belmont Report is that it too uses the principles approach, not that it suggests three instead of four principles. Each of the four groups of principles proposed in this chapter could probably be shrunk to three principles with a little effort and could (more easily) be more finely separated into five or more principles. In the way The Belmont Report individuated its principles, there was no principle of nonmaleficence. And instead of autonomy, it refers to "Respect for Persons." One could say that respect for persons included both autonomy (for persons with capacity) and nonmaleficence (for persons who lack capacity). I choose the four-principle approach as my model for a few reasons, including it is so well known, and one of the primary staff members of The Belmont Report was Tom Beauchamp, who then decided to improve the three principles approach by adding the fourth principle.

Overall, while both sets are perfectly reasonable, the addition of the fourth principle was an improvement. It makes more explicit the importance of getting the voluntary consent of the patient or research participant, rather than appearing to leave that open to the judgment of the doctor or researcher (i.e. to trust the researcher to limit interventions or research to what he or she considers respectful). And adding non-maleficence explicitly recognizes the old Hippocratic adage of "First do no harm," which resonates very deeply with some physicians. Lastly, having four principles allows the balance of two ancient and two modern principles, which seems just right, making explicit that ethics, like medicine and science, ought to be aware of and honor its history yet also be aware that it has made important progress since 500 BCE.

The bottom line for these principles in research ethics for an IRB or ethics review board to consider: for respect for persons, make sure the 'subject' (or participant) not only consented to participation, but understands the risks; make sure the research is worth doing (likely to led to some benefit that is commensurate with the risks being taken) and well designed to accomplish its purpose; and do not take advantage of vulnerable groups who are easier to enroll but whose social group is less likely to gain from the eventual benefits (such as prisoners, the poor, the handicapped, children, or people from developing nations).[10]

On the ethics of research involving animal subjects:
Research using animals as subjects is almost never primarily for benefit of animals, though drugs that result might also end up being used to help other animals. So the usual sense of justice is always violated, using one group (non-human animals) to help another group (human animals)—or else justice simply doesn't apply. And animals can't give consent. So the usual principles are not that helpful. But Beneficence can apply: only do research likely to yield important information, using the right methods and the right number of subjects. And Non-maleficence applies: researchers should try not to harm the animals, don't cause any more pain or suffering than absolutely necessary, and do everything possible to minimize it by using anesthetics and a way to kill them (sacrifice is the common term used) that does not cause them either pain or fear.

The most common rules referred to, more concrete than the mid-level principles of bioethics, are called the three R's: replace, reduce, refine. Replace means do not use animals if you can get valid results without the use of animals. Reduce means use as few animals as possible to get statistically valid results. Refine means use the neurologically simplest species necessary to get your results, i.e. use cell cultures rather than animals when possible, and when you need animals use flies, slugs, snails, fish, frogs, and avoid using mammals whenever possible (and some would say never use primates, or at least never use the great apes). The latter is based on a scientific understanding of what animals can experience, and that more advanced animals deserve greater protection because they are capable of experiencing not just pain, but fear, anxiety, suffering, and even depression (evidenced by objectively observable self-destructive behaviors and objectively measurable vital signs like heart rate and blood pressure).

---

[10]Justice in international research is the most interesting and newest issue to be explored in research ethics. Some worry that if protections aren't set, the kind of double-standard that Tuskegee revealed in the US will simply be outsourced or off-shored, so that researchers from developed nations will treat citizens of the developing world with the same double-standard. See: London AJ. Justice and the human development approach to international research. *Hastings Center Report* 2005; 35(1): 24–37. Lavery J.V., Bandewar S.V., Kimini J., et al. 'Relief of Oppression': An organizational principle for researcher's obligations in the developing world. *BMC Public Health*, 2010; 10: 384–390.

Four Additional Mid-Level Principles for Professionalism (and Professional Integrity)

While the first four principles have been sufficient for hundreds of authors in medicine, dentistry, and nursing, various authors have suggested adding one or two new principles (though it is not always the same one or two principles). There is nothing inherently wrong with any of the suggestions.

Suggestions from various sources have been adapted to produce this extended list of additional principles that have been broadly accepted and used in ethical analyses and justifications in health care.[11] As with the original four, no individual principle can be considered pre-eminent, and this group is best considered only as supplemental principles, only to be added the first four if you find them helpful. In other words, these four principles cannot be considered whatsoever to be potential replacements for the first four principles, and each reader can feel free to use either just the first four, or all eight principles.

Those who think we only need the original four principles usually understand all of the following additional principles as being a part (or implied by) of the principle of beneficence. As with the first four principles, each can be understood as including both an aspirational ideal and (*at least*) a minimal legal duty.

Confidentiality: Always keep information about a patient confidential unless you are required by law to report something. Be careful not to communicate information in a public way, whether in a hall, elevator, or online (e.g., social network sites); *at least* reveal only what is required by law and avoid speculating beyond the evidence you have. It is all too easy to assume the worst about people you do not know (and simultaneously overlook your own flaws) or to get excited (ego involvement) at the prospect of helping authority figures (like hospital administration or the police). One must be consciously aware of such biases and temptations, remain non-judgmental, and carefully avoid using confidential information to enhance one's self-esteem.

Honesty (or in more traditional terminology, Veracity and Fidelity): Always keep your promises and tell the truth. This includes being truthful about errors or mistakes you have made even if they do not lead to any harm or bad outcomes. If the error was not your own, encourage the person who is responsible to tell the

---

[11]The additional professionalism and population-based principles provided in this section have been adapted from various sources, including: P.L. Beemsterboer (2010) *Ethics and Law in Dental Hygiene Practice*, 2nd Edition. St. Louis, MO: Elsevier; essays by Courtney Campbell, Vincent Rogers, Jeffrey Kahn, and Thomas Hasegawa in B.D. Weinstein (ed.) (1993) *Dental Ethics*. Philadelphia, PA: Lea & Febiger Publishing; *Dental Ethics at the Chairside*, 2e, David Ozar and David Sokol, Georgetown (2002). *Case Studies and Nursing Practice: The Ethical Issues* (Prentice-Hall series in the philosophy of medicine) by Andrew Jameton (Feb 1984), *Ethics in Nursing: Cases, Principles, and Reasoning*, 4e. M Benjamin and J Curtis. Oxford (2010), and *Ethics in Nursing Practice*, Sara Fry and Megan-Jane Johnstone, Blackwell (2002), B. Lo *Resolving Ethical Dilemmas: A Guide for Clinicians*, 4th Edition. Baltimore, MD: Wolters Kluwer (2009).

patient. *At the least* do not lie, deceive, mislead, cheat, take credit for the work of others (give due credit to sources and collaborators, and don't allow 'ghost writers'), or give people credit for work that they don't deserve ('guest authorship').

Competence: Always maintain and update your professional knowledge and skills; *at least* defend professional standards by refusing to do things you are not adequately trained to do, referring patients to more qualified professionals, and by reporting incompetent, unethical, or impaired colleagues.

Managing Conflicts of Interest: Clinicians and scientists have a duty to avoid inducements (e.g., salary, bonuses, payments, stock options or investments) that may incentivize overtreatment, influence recommendations, or distort objectivity in research or treatment (e.g. from insurance or pharmaceutical companies); if one doesn't refuse all such inducements, one must *at least* fully and honestly disclose all potential conflicts of interest to funding and regulatory agencies, publishers, patients and research subjects. Some scientists, for example, are concerned that the intrusion of the profit motive and possible short-term financial gains can slowly undermine the more long-term value of basic science.

These four additional principles have more to do with how a professional conducts oneself, or the virtues of the professional, and less to do with the doctor-patient (or dentist-patient, nurse-patient, professional-patient) relationship and their process of shared decision-making. Consequently, these four principles might be referred to as principles of professionalism (in contrast to the first four principles, typically called the four principles of bioethics).

All four of the principles of professionalism can be referred to as a whole as "professional integrity" because the concept of integrity has to do with being well integrated, and, in this case, a professional is thought to have integrity when he or she exemplifies *all* of these qualities. This idea is much the same as the Ancient Greek notion of the unity of the virtues: a person tends to have all of them or none of them. Similarly, these four principles together, rather than any one of them alone, define professional integrity. So while these might be thought of as all a part of Beneficence, they might equally be considered an addition to the principles approach from Aristotelian virtue ethics.

Pearls for professionalism:
Try to like all of your patients and maintain an attitude of "positive regard" towards them, even so-called "noncompliant" ones. Regard them as marching to the beat of a different drummer, as inner-directed (less concerned with/less needy of social acceptance), or as risk takers who put independence before longevity. Think "nonconformist" rather than "noncompliant."

Or, more paradoxically: the best doctors take the worst patients. Sometimes noncompliance is set into motion by poor communication skills on the part of the doctor—authoritarian or arrogant attitudes can trigger some patients to reject your advice. Often noncompliant behavior is the result of physicians' failures. For example, a clinician should prepare a patient for likely side effects so the patient understands they are normal and not a reason to discontinue a medication, or equally common, a clinician must make clear why it is important to finish a course of treatment even if the symptoms disappear after a few days. Otherwise in both scenarios it is hard to put all the blame on the patient for not taking their prescribed medications.

There is also a lesson here for how to treat members of other professions. Good communication skills, demonstrating respect for their knowledge and skills, is vital to effective teamwork. Professionalism should enhance comraderie and ameliorate or eliminate much of the moral distress experienced by members of interprofessional teams.[12]

Four Principles for Public Health

Public health is a very expansive field, including epidemiology, environmental health, occupational health, preventive medicine, health economics, health policy, and more. But there is no reason this approach of developing mid-level principles could not be extended to a health field that focuses on social groups, communities, and populations.

Public Health, more than any other field, deals with conflicts or trade-offs between public and private interests, what's best for the group and what's best for an individual. These questions about what is fair to the individual, and what we as a society can impose on individuals for the greater good, describe much of the field of Public Health Ethics, from vaccinations, to issues surrounding infectious disease (quarantines, partner notification, forced and observed treatment), to business regulations (safety inspections from food and drugs to the workplace, and regulations surrounding the licensing of professions).

Thus Public Health ethics, with its focus on populations, can be seen as refining and defending the importance of the principle of Justice. Just as the four principles that help define professional integrity fill out some of the details of Beneficence, the following four additional principles for Public Health might be considered all to be components of the principle of Justice. But given the complexity of the principle of Justice, and how easy it is for some clinicians to deny its importance, it helps to provide more explanation of what Justice entails. Here then are four principles often cited in the literature of public health ethics.[13]

---

[12]Mitchell C., 1988. Integrity in Interprofessional Relationships. In: Edwards R.B., Glenn C.G. ed., *Bio-ethics.* San Diego: Harcourt Brace Jovanovich. pp. 63–72.

[13]The sources I have found most useful in formulating principles for public health include especially S. Holland (2007) *Public Health Ethics.* Cambridge, MA: Polity Press; and S.S. Coughlin, T.L. Beauchamp and D.L. Weed (2009) *Ethics and Epidemiology*, 2nd Edition. New York: Oxford University Press, and articles by Jonathan Mann, Amartya Sen, Ronald Bayer, Dan Beauchamp, Lawrence Gostin, Larry Churchill, Ruth Faden, and Norman Daniels, reprinted in numerous anthologies.

1. **Procedural Justice**: to require or *at least* encourage (and defend the right to) participation of all affected parties in the decision-making process. Thus if a policy would affect an entire community, all members would have to be informed beforehand and have input into whether to proceed. Or, if decisions of other people could put an individual at risk, then that individual has the right to input on the decision. To work, procedural justice must include transparency: to require truthful information is widely shared and never presented evasively, to hold public meetings and work to build a public consensus.

2. **Least restrictive alternative**: to promote freedom and liberty one must find the way to achieve a goal that does not impose on human rights, or the does so with the least burden possible. John Stuart Mill originally proposed what he called the Harm Principle: Society should allow us to do what we want, even if it is not particularly wise; *(at least)* the only exception when society should limit personal freedom is to prevent harm to others. Deontologists like Kant and Rawls also agree it is vital to protect the rights of the individual, and one can only justify restrictions to protect the rights of other individuals. (An American legal opinion once asserted 'your right to swing your fist ends at the tip of my nose'). This might also be called (more aspirationally or idealistically) the principle of Respect for Human Rights, although that term can be taken to include more (and some would say, too many) ethical claims to ascribe as a responsibility of Public Health.

3. **Precautionary principle**: to maximize human safety when there is some scientific evidence of risk, but it is, as of yet, inconclusive or less than certain. *At the least*, this applies to cases where the damage at risk is severe and cannot be undone. It can be thought of as part of justice in that it would be an injustice if one caused an avoidable harm because of a lack of sufficient evidence of the likelihood or degree of harm. (Colloquially, this can be thought of as the 'better safe than sorry' principle.) It is used more often in laws and regulations in Europe than in the U.S., e.g. restrictions on GMO's and pesticides. In the US, the FDA considers this principle with pharmaceuticals, but we do less testing with chemicals like pesticides, herbicides, cleaners, gasoline additives, or chemicals used in hydraulic fracturing, and hence run more risk of recalls (sometimes after people have been harmed).

4. **Communitarian principle**: Weighs import of social institutions and social connectedness to individual well-being, and hence defines our reciprocal obligations to the group. In the health professions, there has been much recent research into the social determinants of health, showing that genetics and "personal responsibility" *combined* can never be the entire story: we need to live in a society that treats us fairly ("with respect") in order to achieve physical or mental health. Thus our own health and well-being depends largely on how others treat us, hence *at the least* we must reciprocate and contribute to others' well-being. In other words, we each have an ethical duty to agree to our fair share of the burdens or costs required to help correct or diminish unjust constraints in the lives of others, to justify our own benefiting from being a member

of that community. This can include, but is not limited to, universal access to preventive medicine and basic health care.

Taking a cue from Aristotle's humanistic ethics, many commentators want the Communitarian Principle to include whatever is necessary in order to flourish, or achieve one's potential. This might include more than just health care, but extend to education, employment, and other goods necessary for self-respect (although these wouldn't all be the responsibility of health professionals *per se*). And taking a cue from feminist ethics, this may be where women, as a group, must be considered. The *a priori* assumption must be that women deserve the same opportunities as men in terms of health care, education, employment, etc.

This might also be called (again, more aspirationally or idealistically) the principle of social justice, although that term can be taken to include more (and some would say, too many) ethical claims to ascribe as a responsibility of public health. Applying the communitarian principle to economics, one gets what Rawls called The Difference (or Minimax) Principle: inequality (or anything that increases inequality), whether social or economic, is only justified if it benefits the worst-off members of society, by, for example, increasing their opportunities in life or their income. There has been an explosion of important research on the health effects of income inequality in the past decade, lending credence to the idea that the best thing we can do for the health of individuals might be to focus on improving the fairness of the society in which they live.[14]

The Communitarian principle can also be used to defend the physical commons as well as the social commons, that is, to protect the quality of resources we need for a healthy life such as clean air to breath, and clean water to drink, safe food to eat, safe neighborhoods to live in, and even policies to prevent human actions that cause droughts and floods. In all these cases, we need the participation of others in order to achieve these goals for ourselves, and hence we also must be willing to contribute our fair share to others' ability to enjoy "the commons" (or "the common good"). All of these goods are sometimes considered to be within the purview of Public Health.

At the very least, we must avoid the type of injustice called environmental racism, when one community shoulders an undue burden of pollution compared to others because they lack the economic or political power to defend the quality of their neighborhood (habitat). Environmental racism became recognized after protests about PCB dumping in 1982 in Warren County, North Carolina, a predominantly African-American community.[15]

---

[14]For example, see the collection of articles in *Science*, May 23, 2014, special issue on "Haves and Have-nots, the science of inequality" and the book *The Society and Population Health Reader: income inequality and health*, I Kawachi, BP Kennedy, and RG Wilkerson, edd. New Press, Norton Publishers, New York, 1999.

[15]R.D. Bullard, G.S. Johnson, and A.O. Torres ed., *Environmental Health and Racial Equity in the U.S.* APHA Publication, 2011. Robert Bullard, *The Wrong Complexion for Protection*. New York University Press, New York and London, 2012.

Like the original principles, both Utilitarians and Deontologists would be able to provide justifications for each of these four new principles (though not, of course, the same justifications). Each, in other words, can be seen as both logical (implied by such laws as logical consistency and the law of non-contradiction) as well as scientifically supported by the evidence. And, also like the original four principles, these principles are independent, meaning one must consider them all, and in some cases they may come into conflict with each other. Thus, they too have a solid claim to being of very wide acceptability and usefulness, so long as one doesn't mistakenly think they make cases simple, or always yield a single correct answer. They will, in other words, help us better understand a difficult or complex case and avoid many ethical mistakes that come from oversimplification.

One final observation: these four principles for public health might be thought of as revisions of Autonomy, Beneficence, Non-maleficence, and Justice, in that order, revised to apply to populations rather than individuals—whether clinicians or patients, scientists or research participants. So there is still room for a person to insist that one only needs the original four principles. This may come down to the classic distinction from Sir Isaiah Berlin of hedgehogs and foxes, or lumpers and splitters. Readers should each be free to choose the system that they find most helpful. For some too many principles will be distracting, while for others allowing greater plasticity in the meaning of a principle will be confusing.

Chapter 5
Instructional Materials for Students and Teachers

Instructional Materials for Students: A Case Analysis Method to Write Short-Answer 'Free-Response' Questions (FRQs), Essays, and Papers with Valid Ethical Arguments and Sound Conclusions (Including a Grading Matrix for Teachers and Students)

Now we can offer a model of how to approach an ethical problem and produce an ethical argument, that is, make a well justified or sound recommendation in a case analysis, for an essay on a test or for a paper in a course.

1. What are the facts? What more do you need to know? Good ethics begins with good facts: First collect all the pertinent scientific, clinical, and population data; then the perspective of all stakeholders, whether they are neighborhood residents, patients, or research participants. You can only accurately and fairly identify the ethical issues after this process. If there is important information lacking, identify what else you need to know before making any judgments. Then (and only then) you should identify the ethical issues.

    Here casuistry or narrative ethics can play an essential role in describing an ethical process for case analysis ("casuistry" is derived from "cases"). To do it well requires attention to details, sensitivity to seek out and listen to people who may be marginalized, and is more 'bottom-up' than mere 'logical deduction' from either mid-level Principles or general theories like Kant's Categorical Imperative (which, it must be added, was never the suggested approach of Beauchamp and Childress).

2. What are the ethical issues? Identify the ethical issues and outline all the options: Identify every reasonable alternative course of action, and the most likely outcome of each. (This is where one sees the value of Utilitarianism; one cannot ignore the consequences of the choices—the consequences of your acts count.) Some choices may only address one issue, or even make other issues worse. So try to address all of the issues you identified. Identifying only one issue or option

© The Author(s) 2016
J.P. Spike and R. Lunstroth, *A Casebook in Interprofessional Ethics*,
SpringerBriefs in Ethics, DOI 10.1007/978-3-319-23769-5_5

usually indicates a weakness in the analysis. Sometimes each person involved in the case has a different recommendation on how to resolve the issue.

3. What are the arguments? How do the various principles (or theories) apply? Construct ethical arguments: Outline the pros and cons for each option you identified, using the Principles outlined above, as well as experience from previous cases, applicable Professional Codes of Ethics and Statements ("white papers," guidelines) from recognized professional organizations, hospital or state or federal policies, state and federal laws, and international organizations like the World Health Organization. All of these can be sources of helpful conceptual frameworks that contribute to the sophistication of the reasoning process and its ethical content.

"Dilemma" means there are at least two options with good supporting arguments. Not every case presents a dilemma once it has been analyzed, but every case has legitimate ethical issues. To be more complete, you can ask yourself how each of the principles might advise you to act in the situation. If you end up with two or more good (but imperfect) choices, it is not a fault of your analysis; it just means you have a genuine dilemma on your hands. And if you don't end up with a dilemma, you will still benefit from the identification and clarification of the ethical issues involved.

4. What is the best choice? Present and defend one decision: Use your judgment to determine the ethically best option, i.e. answer the questions "What is the best thing to do?" or "What are your obligations, as a professional and as a citizen?" Consider which choice seems to be supported by the most principles and policies; likewise which option will satisfy the most stakeholders (or the persons with the most at stake), or if one person (or profession) has more right to be the decision-maker.

Just as a math or chemistry teacher won't take an answer without showing your work, since it might just be a lucky guess, the same is true for ethics. You must explain why you made the choice you have made. Different principles can lead to different decisions, and good judgment (practical wisdom, *phronesis*) can depend on your level of experience, imagination, critical thinking, and problem solving.

5. How will you proceed? Recommend a course of action, anticipate arguments against it, discuss what it might take to negotiate a resolution and build a consensus, and document the plan. Acting with integrity and idealism is the goal, rather than expediency. Don't be reticent; keep in mind that taking no action has the same effect as giving tacit approval of the *status quo*. In this final step, strength of character (e.g. the courage to raise controversial issues in a risk-averse organization) can become an important factor.

Pearl:
In ethics, you've got to have a heart, but you've also got to have a spine.—
Steve Miles, physician, ethicist, and activist.

Negotiating professional differences will be at the heart of many interprofessional conflicts and, at the same time, will hold the key to their successful resolution. The case commentary, in these instances, should recognize this and include procedural guidance rather than merely name one or more general principles or claims that might seem to 'solve' a problem but in fact may be likely to fail, or to feel like it is forcing a solution on the case from the outside (using authority rather than ethics to resolve differences).

As with many other models that appear to invoke steps or stages, there is no restriction on the order. Step one takes the most time, and no matter how the case progresses you will commonly find you need to go back and collect more information, and then reconsider the other steps. The back-and-forth process resembles what philosopher John Rawls called "reflective equilibrium."

If you follow this general process, you should arrive at carefully thought out conclusions with strong ethical justifications. For a short-answer free-response question (one paragraph) you will only need a sentence or two that addresses each element. For a short essay (e.g. one or two pages) students should write one paragraph that addresses each of the five questions, in order to make sure their answer is complete. For a longer research paper (perhaps 5–10 pages), that would be an excellent outline to begin with, followed by seeking references and filling out your reasoning process. The research will naturally involve more time and effort, finding books and articles already written on the topic, and assessing their relevance. For these papers one might find the position statements or 'white papers' of various professional health care organizations most helpful—getting something more specific and grounded in practice rather than something more general, abstract, or philosophical. Longer papers also allow you to more fully consider different alternatives, and explain why you chose the one you did.

Those essays or paragraphs would yield a well-organized and reasoned answer. While two people might still arrive at different conclusions, you will have all the grounds you need for comparing notes and judging which conclusion has the best support. And even if you don't come to an agreement, it will no longer be a 'mere' difference of opinion: you will be at least part of the way down the road to establishing a socially and ethically agreeable consensus to resolve the problem presented by the case. This process, followed by scores of people and organizations over a period of many years, is how ethics makes progress.

On Grading:

Sometimes it helps students to know how your analysis might be graded. In the world of teaching, faculty are often encouraged to use a grading rubric or matrix to improve the objectivity or fairness of grading papers. Rubrics can be validated by having two or more teachers grade the same papers and see if they result in the same grades. A typical scheme might be to assign to the answers of each of the five above questions a score of 0 (step skipped, overlooked, not addressed—or occasionally just plain wrong, sarcastic, or unethical or unprofessional), 1 (adequate, acceptable, average, but demonstrates minimal effort, uninspiring, hasty work, done quickly, only one element or option identified, not complete), or 2 (complete, well thought out, careful, clearly expressed, maybe even surprising, original—reflecting serious effort).

This would make a grade range of 0–10, a simple scoring system like the Apgar score in the clinical world that gives a quick but accurate evaluation, with "10" being an excellent paper (for a newborn: thriving, pink or full of color (not pallid, gray or chalky), all four limbs wiggling, and lets out a clear cry with its first breath). Anything below a "5" means a tragedy, either initiating a resuscitation effort ("Code Blue"), or calling the morgue.

Most people will get a 1 or 2 on most answers, so the normal range for most grades will be from 5 to 10, and there will be a clear difference between any 5 or 6 and any 8 or 9. Grade-watchers ('gunners') may think of a 9 as an A, 8 as a B, 7 as a C, and 6 as a D. A score of 5 by a student who didn't take the assignment very seriously can still be brought up to a passing average if the next 10-point assignment improves to an 8. So when possible, it always helps pedagogically if there are a few assignments for students, so they can document their improvement.

To help students improve their grades, they might be given this rubric in advance, and told to be sure to address each of the five elements.

Instructional Materials for Ethics Facilitators: Can Ethics Be Taught?

An Excursion in Socratic Pedagogy

Socrates also famously asked whether ethics can be taught. It can. But not by rote memorization or indoctrination, for that would be (at best) morality, the result of unreflective internalization of beliefs given by an outside authority and internalized without being tested for their truth or validity.

The best way to teach ethics is to provide cases that interest students because they represent situations they know they will face themselves. This gives students a chance to express their opinion, and hear the opinions of other students as well as respected experts. In such disciplined discussions they each must find justifications for their views (or realize their opinion may be unjustifiable). Learning ethics is not a matter of memorizing facts, it is a matter of challenging opinions, wrestling intellectually with humanistic issues, and then maturing. Done well, it is active, interactive, enjoyable, and ends with personal development. (This pedagogical advice holds as well for science: a scientist is not someone who has memorized the content of current textbooks, but who learns science through inquiry, and as a result can formulate and test his or her own hypotheses.)

If you aren't usually an ethics teacher, you may be worried about being asked to incorporate this into your course, and might want some pointers on how to help students enjoy this material and learn from it. Like most teaching, especially in the humanities, it is important to give students time to think and express opinions. This means keeping any one student from dominating, even if (or especially if) they know more than the others, and encourage quiet students to speak up. Quiet kids can have a lot to say, but just be reticent about speaking up, fearful of being wrong. But they often have something to contribute that could help the group. To encourage this, sometimes a facilitator will have to direct a question directly to them, and tolerate long silences before allowing anyone else to speak up.[1]

Early stage or naive professional students may want black and white answers, right or wrong. But they will find the class more interesting if they participate in a group process. Once they see some of the conflicting alternatives between narrow self-interest or being idealistic, and about the possible consequences, and some of the rules or principles you might follow, you should be able to generate a messy— but realistic–debate.

More mature students will know more of the relevant information. You can offer some of that from your own experience, but don't allow that too often or you will encourage them to just look to you for answers. Have them look their questions up in class, or assign relevant background articles as class preparation. If at the end of the class or module they realize they can't just jump to a conclusion in ethics, and it isn't just opinion, and other people see things differently, and they must defend or justify their opinion, then you have accomplished one of the major goals of ethics education.

If you have also given them a sense of the most common issues they will have to deal with in their future career, you have provided them a great service–even if they don't fully appreciate it until those events occur to them in real life. And you will have accomplished both of the major goals of ethics education!

One final reason to teach ethics is that it is an expectation of society, part of the social contract that creates a profession, which members of the profession must understand and agree to follow. So one purpose of this book is to inform students of the expectations society has of them, which they tacitly agree to meet once they enter one of the health care professions. This topic can be introduced, for example, by reading and discussing the Codes of Ethics for various professions, often a surprisingly informative introduction to the topic. Even when teaching students from other professions than your own, it can be interesting to ask if there should be any differences, and why?[2,3]

---

[1]See book by Susan Cain, *Quiet: The Power of Introverts in a World That Can't Stop Talking*, Broadway Books, New York, 2012.

[2]I suggest reading two Codes, just for comparison. One might be "Medical Professionalism in the New Millennium: A Physician Charter" (*Ann Intern Med* 2002:136:243–246), because of its international recognition. It was developed by the American Board of Internal Medicine, the American College of Physicians, and the European Federation of Internal Medicine.

[3]Hull R.T. Ethics: codes or no codes? *Kans Nurse.* 1980 Nov;55(10):8, 18–21.

But the method is not to make pronouncements about what students must do, but to offer them some interesting cases to discuss in class, or small groups, or to analyze in papers, in order to develop and test and refine their ability to think more clearly about ethical problems. Thus students will, it is hoped, grow from having less reflective, less tested moral responses to having a more reflective and sophisticated understanding of the ethical consensus (and how it developed) by treading that ground themselves. The current new term for such personal growth is "identity formation" and so this casebook can be considered a pedagogical tool to promote professional identity formation for the health professions.[4]

The cases in this book are presented without providing any 'answer.' But that doesn't mean there isn't any right answer. Indeed, saying in ethics there is no right answer is a common pedagogical mistake. A facilitator might be tempted to say that in class to demonstrate humility, and to encourage students to speak up. But it can be misunderstood by students as admitting the kind of subjectivity (all opinions are equal) that you are trying to get students to outgrow. Students must be assured that in ethics there are some important lessons to be learned, some important guidelines to follow, and some common mistakes to avoid. That is the general attitude towards ethics for facilitators to project: this is very _useful_ information if you are to provide effective patient care, conduct ethical scientific research, or analyze ethical issues in public health policy. In other words, the group *is* in search of answers, carefully articulated and justified. So you do not wish to accidentally imply that there are no answers, and let some students conclude ethics is not helpful.

The primary job of the ethics facilitator is to keep the discussion going. When a student shares an opinion, thank him for sharing it, and ask for his rationale for his position. After groups do this a few times, criteria of valid conclusions will emerge, roughly as follows: *Were each of the value conflicts addressed? Did the argument consider all parties affected by the action and potential consequences to each? Were all relevant facts considered? Were the professional obligations discussed in terms of widely accepted principles?*

Some other good follow-up questions: Focus on action, i.e., ask: *What would you do or say to the people who are in this situation?* Question information and challenge assumptions, i.e., ask: *How confident are you that what someone told you is true? Do you know that?* Do you know that? Look for useful analogies (and misleading analogies), i.e., ask: *How does this situation compare to others you've seen? The tone should be one of seriousness and urgency: you are asking the student how to deal with a problem that he or she is very likely to face someday.*

---

[4]There is a separate literature on what makes a profession: for example, clear training requirements and/or exams for licensing, and following a Code of Ethics or professional behavior, and a disciplinary process for violating it, and in exchange legal rights to do some things that no one else is allowed to do, and getting paid for your skills. One might say that not violating the Code of your profession is a minimal standard, and that ethics is the discipline that allows you to contemplate a higher standard, an ideal to aspire to, rather than the low level of morality represented by just following rules or 'compliance.' See John Kultgen. *Ethics and Professionalism.* U of Penn Press, Philadelphia, 1988.

Encourage diverse opinions and be sure that all important points of view are represented. When they are not, try to get participants to develop them by asking questions like: *How might the patient view this problem?* Or: *What arguments might the family make?* Or: *What are the potential long-term consequences of that?* That's better than "playing devil's advocate" (taking a contrary position yourself).

> ### In sum, effective ethics discussion facilitators follow these guidelines:
>
> 1. *Effective ethics facilitators are willing to explore areas outside their own area of expertise because they are not there as experts.*
> 2. *Effective ethics facilitators keep the discussion going and do not provide answers. Answers stop discussions. Get the group interested in searching for reasons for their proposed answers.*
> 3. *Socratic teaching advice: no matter what students say, respond with a question until they figure out a better answer for themselves. Says Harvard Law Professor Alan Dershowitz: "I don't answer questions. I question answers."*
> 4. *Effective ethics facilitators establish an environment where it's safe not to know. Tell students it is acceptable to say "I don't know," but it is even better to say "I will look it up and report my results to the group by email" (or at the next class meeting). You can model that behavior by admitting you don't have the answer to a question, and ask one of the students to look up to see what their own professional society has to say on the topic and report back to you (and the group).*

The issues raised by good cases are exciting enough to provoke discussion, and in the course of the discussion, the initial outlines of a consensus will often emerge. Participating in this process is enough to help students understand what ethics is, where it comes from, and why it is a legitimate and valuable pursuit. Most importantly for facilitators, getting your students to recognize issues as ethical, that is, realizing that the fundamental question in some interesting and controversial cases is ethical in nature is half the battle. Once they understand the questions correctly, the search for the correct types of answers should become a willing journey of inquiry based learning.

Chapter 6
Cases

This chapter offers 30 cases for discussion. Each one involves professionals from different fields confronting a shared situation, with the intent of provoking a constructive dialogue about what each professional can contribute to reaching an ethical solution. Some cases only involve two professions, but many involve three or more different professions.

Each case is introduced with a brief synopsis of the issues it raises and the professions most likely to be involved, and is followed by a few questions for students to discuss, whether in a face-to-face classroom setting or in an online discussion. The cases can also be used as essay or paper topic assignments by faculty.

Browse through the following 30 cases. We hope you find many of the cases interesting, even some cases outside of your profession. The effect, we hope, will be to buttress the central claim of this book which is that ethics is an important common ground for all of the health professions. Furthermore, when we recognize that our professions converge upon a common goal we will find less conflict and more pleasure in working together.

All the cases were first drafted by one member of our Campus Wide Ethics Program, then discussed by the entire CWEP group, and revised by the original author. The entire set of cases then had significant editing by the book editor (JS) and by Rebecca Lunstroth to give them greater consistency in style, length, and organization. After the title of each case the professional fields involved in the case are identified, and after each case a few questions are suggested to stimulate discussion.

One final observation about the selection of cases to note is both a strength and weakness: our cases are the result of a democratic process. The choices of working professionals in many fields have a distinct advantage over any one person trying to identify the issues in many different professions (many not his or her own). Still, it must be admitted, there is no systematic process behind the selection of topics— what you have is the result of over a year of meetings. If the cases miss some important topics you, the reader were hoping to be included, I have two suggestions. First, write up your own case for your teaching, and use only those in this book you find helpful. Second, please contact the editor of this book to make suggestions for cases and topics to be included in future editions.

© The Author(s) 2016

J.P. Spike and R. Lunstroth, *A Casebook in Interprofessional Ethics*, SpringerBriefs in Ethics, DOI 10.1007/978-3-319-23769-5_6

These were the original members of the Campus-Wise Ethics Program (CWEP) at UTH, who wrote the first draft of these cases:

Director:
Jeffrey Spike, Ph.D.
Graduate School of Biomedical Sciences:
William Seifert, Jr., Ph.D.
Rebecca Lunstroth, J.D., M.A.
Medical School:
Eugene Boisaubin, M.D.
Nathan Carlin, Ph.D.
School of Biomedical Informatics:
Jonathan Ishee, J.D., M.P.H., M.S., L.L.M.
School of Dentistry:
Richard Bebermeyer, D.D.S., M.B.A.
Catherine Flaitz, D.D.S., M.S.
School of Nursing:
Joan Engebretson, Dr.P.H., R.N., AHN-BC
Dorothy Otto, M.S.N., Ed.D., R.N.
Cathy Rozmus, Ph.D., R.N.
School of Public Health:
Stephen Linder, Ph.D.
Cynthia Chappell, Ph.D.

Outline of Cases by Profession Involved

Profession	Relevant cases
Biomedical sciences	3, 5, 6, 7, 8, 26
Chiropractic	24
Clinical psychology	2, 21, 22
Clinical social work	12
Dentistry	10, 11, 15, 16, 18, 19, 20, 25
Dental assistant	10, 16, 17, 18, 19
Dental hygiene	10, 16
Health informatics	1, 2, 3, 9, 12
Medicine	1, 2, 3, 4, 5, 6, 7, 8, 9, 10, 11, 12, 13, 14, 15, 17, 18, 20, 21, 22, 23, 24, 25, 27, 28, 29, 30
Nurse practitioner	18, 25

(continued)

(continued)

Profession	Relevant cases
Nursing	1, 2, 4, 7, 10, 11, 12, 13, 14, 15, 16, 17, 20, 21, 22, 23, 24, 27, 28, 29, 30
Pharmacy	24, 25, 30
Physician assistant	17, 18, 25
Public health	4, 5, 13, 14, 15, 19, 20, 26
Social work	2, 11, 21, 22, 27
Translational medicine	5, 26

Case 1: The Limitations of Electronic Health Records (EHRs), Decision-Support, and Financial Conflicts of Interest

Relevant Professions: Health Informatics, Medicine, Nursing

Issues: The limitations of EMRs, and Conflict of interest.

Why this is important: The recent push for widespread adoption of Health Informatics raises significant concerns related to the safety and oversight of electronic health records (EHRs) and HIT (health information technology).

The Case: This year Hope Hospital spent Fifty Million Dollars ($50,000,000) to acquire Protogram, an electronic health record (EHR). Protogram t has a full featured suite of patient care and decision making tools including clinical decision support (CDS), drug-drug interaction checker, and computerized physician order entry (CPOE). This system was designed by Judy Green, Owner of Protogram Software, LLC and member of Hope's Board of Directors.

As the Chief Informatics Officer of the hospital you feel confident that this new system will improve overall patient care, however you have become concerned with reports from the medical staff that there is an issue with the drug-drug interaction checker. This issue only arises when one particular combination of drugs are prescribed. These two medications should not be prescribed together as they cause severe adverse reactions in patients up to and including death. The EHR should alert users to this potentially deadly combination at the time the medication is ordered but the system seems to only catch and alert users 95 % of the time. You have alerted Judy, the board, the employed physicians and hospital staff to this issue on numerous occasions and Judy has indicated that they are aware of the issue and are working to fix it. Six (6) months have gone by and still no update has been released. The hospital has had too many "close calls" to count, as physicians become more and more reliant on CDS and the drug-drug interaction functionality of the EHR.

Today, the Hope's CEO stopped by your office to inform you that the hospital's board has approved the purchase and donation of Protogram t to non-hospital based primary care providers who have regular and courtesy privileges at the Hospital. During your discussion with the CEO on this issue you mention that you think this is a bad idea since a software fix has not been released, and even if the hospital alerted the PCPs to the issue it would not prevent future events from occurring. Upon hearing this, the CEO states that, due to the confidentiality provisions of the software agreement, the hospital cannot inform anyone other than hospital employees or the vendor of any issues related to the software. Additionally, the CEO states that failure to abide by the confidentiality provision will nullify the agreement with Protagram and subject the hospital to a costly lawsuit (costing between forty and seventy million dollars), cause significant issues with the hospital's board, and the termination of any employee(s) who released the information.

Questions:

1. What should the hospital CEO do?
2. Should the hospital's potential financial liabilities offset the potential harms to patients, even if the harms aren't likely to occur? How much say should belong to the CFO rather than the CEO?
3. What should you, the Chief Informatics Officer say to the CEO and do you have an obligation to report this to the Board?

Case 2: Preserving Privacy and Confidentiality with Electronic Health Records

Relevant Professions: Health Informatics, Medicine, Nursing, Clinical Psychology, Social Work

Issues: The tension between patient safety and patient privacy and the role technology plays in meeting your professional obligations to each of these; data segmentation; psychiatric history.

Why this is important: The recent push for patient centered HIT applications raises significant concerns related to the safety and oversight of such systems.

The case: Boogle, a global software company and large internet search website recently released PHR Vault, a software platform that allows patients to download their medical information into a personal health record (PHR) and electronically share that information with health providers who use an electronic health record (EHR) that is connected to the local health information exchange (HIE). This information is provided seamlessly to the provider and is automatically inserted into the provider's EHR. Boogle recently released an update to PHR Vault that allows patients to choose which PHR data they would like to share with specific healthcare providers.

Mary-Lou Smith a 40 year old female patient, recently came to your office to be seen for depression. Her regular PCP (primary care physician) is a medical school classmate of yours. Mary-Lou is the Executive Vice President of Excel Energy, a Fortune 100 company. During the visit she mentions that she does not want the reason for the visit recorded in her chart since a diagnosis of depression could threaten her job. You determine that she does, in fact, suffer from depression and prescribe Zoloft. Mary-Lou forbids you from disclosing the visit to any other providers, pays cash, and does not use her health insurance to cover the cost of the visit. Furthermore, she gets her Zoloft filled at a local independently owned pharmacy paying cash.

Recently, it has come to your attention that Mary-Lou didn't tell her regular PCP that she is taking Zoloft and has set up her PHR to prevent sharing this information with him. You are concerned that failure to share this information may be detrimental to her health and cause a potential adverse reaction to any drugs that are subsequently prescribed by her PCP.

Questions:

1. How do you balance a patient's privacy needs with your duty to ensure their health and safety?
2. What is the proper role of technology and is there ever risk introduced by overreliance on technology?
3. There is a long tradition of keeping patient's psychiatric care in a separate file to protect their privacy. Should HIT allow this to continue, in the name of patient's rights, or should the technology be used to improve communication between providers and insurance companies?

Case 3: Privacy in the Age of Patient-Driven Websites

Relevant Professions: Health Informatics, Medicine, Biomedical Sciences

Issues: Privacy and Technology.

Why this is important: The recent push for widespread adoption of health informatics raises significant concerns related to the privacy and security of health information.

The Case: Having become disillusioned with your research job at big pharma you take a job at a local research institution dedicated to the research and cure of rare diseases. After starting your new job you learn of a new website, "Patients Like You", where individuals with rare diseases can share personal and clinical information with others in an attempt to improve the lives of similarly situated people. To facilitate this exchange of information, "Patients Like You" has created a platform for collecting and sharing outcome-based data with other patients. You have heard that many patients with rare conditions use the website to talk to each other and exchange information about the various available treatments.

Upon creating a member account, users agree to the terms of the site's privacy statement which grants the site the unrestricted ability to use the data in the research and treatment of the disease. Having seen that the site currently has 10,000 members sharing data on the disease you are researching, you contact it to see if they will provide you with a list of local physicians who are treating this patient population to ascertain whether they might want to participate in an upcoming research trial. "Patients Like You" informs you that while they cannot provide you with a list of local physicians, they can provide you with detailed patient data (including personally identifiable information) on the 10,000 patients for a small fee of $100.00 per patient.

Questions:

1. In what situation would it be appropriate for you to receive the data held by "Patients Like You"?
2. Does it matter that the site is charging for the data?
3. Would the situation be different if the patient expressly authorized the site to provide the data to anyone requesting the information? Does checking a box on the website legally suffice as "expressly authorizing"? And should it?
4. Is there anything you would want to know before recommending a decision?

Case 4: Workplace Wellness Programs and Health Disparities

Relevant Professions: Medicine, Nursing, Public Health

Issues: Health promotion in the workplace; Health disparities.

Why this is important: The Affordable Care Act contains provisions incentivizing employers to adopt workplace wellness programs however, to what extent should an employer be involved in the health of its workforce?

The case: Obesity, hypertension, and diabetes have reached epidemic proportions throughout the United States. The Affordable Care Act (ACA) recognizes the impact these epidemics have on rising health care costs and includes provisions to incentivize healthy behaviors through workplace wellness programs. Although the Health Insurance Portability and Accountability Act (HIPAA) of 1996 prohibits charging subscribers a higher premium based on health status, it is legal to give premium discounts or rebates to those who adhere to programs of health promotion and disease prevention.

You are the medical director for a Fortune 500 company and the board of directors has requested that you design a wellness program that would ultimately reduce the incidence of obesity and diabetes among the company's 30,000 employees. The first thing you did was analyze the demographic information for your urban work force. The results were revealing but not unexpected: those employees who earned less than $40,000 a year had significantly worse health than those who earned more than $40,000 a year. The data was further bifurcated for the lowest wage earners. As expected, health care spending was proportionate to these findings.

Questions:

1. What is the best way to incentivize your workforce to adopt and maintain healthy lifestyles without overtly singling out your low wage earners?
2. Some executive 'gold plans' include not just gym memberships, but personal trainers. Should you add that to your low wage earners' benefits?
3. What are the benefits and burdens for companies who choose to intervene in the health of their employees?

Case 5: Conducting Human Subject Research Abroad: Whose Standards?

Relevant Professions: Biomedical Science, Translational Science, Medicine, Public Health

Issue: Protection of Human Subjects.

Why this is important: Increasingly biomedical research is being conducted in developing (resource poor) countries. No matter where you live, you may have an opportunity to be involved in research in other countries.

The case: Aragen, a UK-based company has developed a vaccine against HIV that appears promising. Animal studies were very successful. Phase I and phase II trials demonstrated that the vaccine was remarkably safe and it produced significant antibody levels in essentially all of the volunteers. The company now wishes to begin phase III trials in Guatemala where previous surveillance studies revealed a very high incidence of HIV. Such a study could be completed in two years. The Guatemalan government has expressed interest in having the study conducted and begins negotiations with Aragen. The vaccine, which is specifically directed against the strain in the Guatemalan population, will be provided free by Aragen. The company will cover the cost of conducting the study, which will be carried out by the Guatemala Vaccine Institute. In addition to the study costs, the company will provide all the laboratory equipment necessary to conduct the studies, ten computers for the Institute, and two vehicles to visit the study sites. The company agrees that if the vaccine proves effective it will be given free of charge to the affected population of the city at no cost to the country for five years.

In designing the Phase III study the sponsor Aragen proposes a randomized double blind prospective study with one group receiving the test vaccine and the other group receiving a placebo. All potential participants will be tested for HIV prior to being enrolled in the study. If they are HIV + they will be referred to one of the municipal hospitals of the Guatemala Corporation. Further, any research subject who converts to HIV + during the study will be randomized—half will be referred to one of the Municipal Corporation hospitals to be treated by the standard method in Guatemala, which does not include retroviral drugs, including AZT, or any protease inhibitors. The other half will not be told of their HIV status to measure whether the vaccine has any impact on the disease as suggested by animal models. If there is any change in the standard therapy recommended by the government, any previous or future seroconvert or will be switched to this therapy. Due to the AIDS epidemic, the Guatemalan government has proposed making the vaccine mandatory, however, once enrolled the subjects can withdraw at any time. The Municipal Corporation will continue to provide treatment for the patient's lifetime.

Questions:

1. When, if ever, can the cost difference of conducting studies in developing countries be ethically justified?
2. What are the ethical standards for conducting research? Are they the same in all countries? Should a study like this meet the standards of the U.S. or Guatemala or both?
3. You are the chairman of an IRB in a developing county tasked with evaluating this protocol. What questions would you ask? Do you need any additional information? What would you advise and why?

Case 6: Authorship and Clinical Equipoise

Relevant Professions: Medicine and Biomedical Science

Issues: Authorship, Placebo controlled studies, Children in research, Financial conflict of interest, Research in developing (resource poor) countries, and Identifying when parents are being coerced to give consent.

Why this is important: One of the most common complaints among researchers has to do with who gets (or doesn't get) authorship credits of a paper. Secondly, in randomized clinical trials it is assumed that there is clinical equipoise; that one intervention isn't better than the other.

The case: Dr. Stanford is a scientist who has been conducting research for the past ten years on genetic defects in the biosynthesis of biopterin, the absence of which leads to a severe type of phenylketonuria (PKU). Most forms of PKU are effectively treated through diet, but not in this instance. Left untreated, this genetic defect leads to cognitive disability and motor neuron disease. Dr. Stanford has found a method by which synthetic biopterin can be efficiently transported across the blood brain barrier in laboratory rats. He contacted his university's patent office immediately after the discovery 4 years ago. At that same time he contacted Dr. Peterson, an esteemed pediatric neurologist at the university to ensure that his research would be transferable to her patient population. Dr. Peterson fully endorsed Dr. Stanford's research and told him that she would like to collaborate. Dr. Stanford prepared a manuscript documenting his laboratory findings and sent it to Dr. Peterson for review. Dr. Peterson was upset that she wasn't listed as a co-author.

Drs. Stanford and Peterson recently concluded a Phase I trial of the drug in Honduras and Mexico and are currently working on a multi-centered Phase II protocol. Additionally, they have formed a spin-off company with the biotechnology firm DDX which will hopefully produce and market the new drug once it receives FDA approval. The Phase II protocol (double-blinded placebo-controlled) will include Dr. Peterson's patient population. Dr. Peterson is privy to information about the drug thus, she wants to give her patients the study drug and somehow arrange to give a placebo to a colleague's patients. She approaches Dr. Stanford with this arrangement.

Questions:

1. What is the ethical standard that defines who should be listed as an author of a paper? The International Committee of Medical Journal Editors (ICMJE) has published guidelines for authorship.
2. How should patients be recruited for a new study? Can a doctor leading the study recruit her own patients, and what protections should be built into such a study protocol?
3. Is it ethical for the researchers to own a company (or stock in a company) that will make money if the research proves successful?
4. When, (if ever) is a placebo controlled study ethical when studying a serious disease with irreversible consequences for children?

Case 7: When Professional Identity Conflicts with Research

Relevant Professions: Medicine, Biomedical Sciences and Nursing

Issue: Nurses as patient advocates; Executing research protocols; Alternative and complementary medicine.

Why this is important: Principal Investigator's responsibility to a research protocol may conflict with the normal fiduciary duty to the patient's best interest. Nursing staff taking care of a patient may also be caught in this bind, even though they are not involved in the research.

The case: Dr. Fellmann is a neuroscientist who has been studying acute anxiety in primates. He has developed a combined therapy using benzodiazepine and a newly developed, fast-acting anxiolytic agent called AA-1202. Use of the combined therapy in primates has been so successful that it was patented. Dr. Fellmann is collaborating with a cardiac surgeon, Dr. Earl, because they believe that this combined therapy might be beneficial for patients who are about to undergo surgery. They recently concluded a Phase 1 study testing its safety and a multi-center Phase 2 clinical trial has been approved by the University's IRB.

The Phase 2 clinical trial is a double-blind, placebo-controlled protocol that will include two different dosages of the combined therapy. They will recruit patients who are scheduled for cardiac surgery. As part of the protocol, patients are admitted the afternoon prior to surgery and are given the study drug or placebo at 7:00 P.M. Vital signs and pain levels are monitored hourly. All subjects are administered an anxiety scale instrument at the time the drug is administered as well the next morning.

One of the floor nurses, Ms. Patel, has a great deal of experience with surgical patients. She has worked the cardiac pre-op. floor for 15 years and frequently uses a mindfulness meditation technique to ease patients' fears prior to surgery. Clinical experience has taught her that patients who use this technique seem to be less anxious prior to their surgical procedures. One evening, Dr. Earl noticed that Ms. Patel was teaching this technique to one of his patients who as scheduled for cardiac surgery in the morning and who was enrolled in the Phase 2 trial. Dr. Earl asks to see Ms. Patel in the hall where he explains that since this patient was enrolled in the clinical trial for the pre-surgical anti-anxiety medication she should refrain from using the meditation technique.

Questions:

1. Do you think Dr. Earl is justified in asking Ms. Patel to refrain from using a mindfulness meditation technique with the patients enrolled in the clinical trial? Why or why not?
2. Nurse Patel has an obligation to offer help her patients. Does she have a similar obligation to follow the orders of an attending physician?
3. How should you rectify the conflict at hand?

Case 8: When Experimental Therapies Need to Be Tested

Relevant Professions: Medicine, Biomedical Science

Issues: Experimental therapies and when experimental therapies should undergo research.

Why this is important: Many ideas are touted in the popular press and social media with little scientific support. Some are even advertised by "real doctors." Patients often want information about such treatments and may even be anxious to try them.

The case: The chief executive officer of a large, multi-national engineering firm has suffered with chronic back pain for years. Recently his orthopedic surgeon suggested an injection of his own stem cells (which had earlier been removed from fat in his body and cultured in a lab) to address the ongoing problem. Stem cell injections are not licensed for use by the Food and Drug Administration but there has been quite a bit of federally approved research in recent years, from heart disease to brain injury to multiple sclerosis. The therapy performed on the CEO was until recently only available overseas and this was the first time the orthopedic surgeon gave a patient an injection of his own stem cells. Following the procedure and its positive results, a stem cell bank was formed with the CEO's orthopedic surgeon as a co-owner. It has collected stem cells from roughly 70 prospective patients since it launched in August and has procedures scheduled to re-inject the cells as therapy in 30 of those patients.

A number of physicians at the hospital in which the stem cell infusions are scheduled to be performed are concerned about the safety and efficacy of the procedures and believe that they should be reviewed by the hospital's institutional review board (IRB).

Questions:

1. To what extent should physicians be able to use off-label or unproven treatments? Do doctors have the right to try new things so long as the patient consents?
2. In what instances should novel approaches first undergo clinical trials before they are approved for wide-spread us?
3. Is the hospital's IRB the appropriate forum to review these procedures?
4. What is research? Does it include trying novel or innovative treatments on a patient or a few patients, does it require writing a protocol and following it in order to collect data and test a hypothesis?

Case 9: When Practice Guidelines Conflict with Professional Authority

Relevant Professions: Health Informatics, Medicine

Issues: Profit motives and Electronic Medical Records (EMR).

Why this is important: While clinicians are afraid that decision-making software built into EMRs limit their professional authority they are also free to exercise their clinical judgement. It is not clear whether ignoring guidelines results in better care or higher prices.

The case: The Internal Medicine Group of Houston (IMGH) is comprised of 20 general practitioners and 10 sub-specialists. The group implemented a robust electronic health record (EHR) 6 months ago and was recently certified as a top tier medical home. The practice is also a Medicare Advantage IPA (Independent Practice Association) that holds a risk contract for a portion of its Medicare population whereby they are both provide the care and act as the insurance provider. The EHR helps facilitate patients who have chronic diseases and ensures that each and every patient is provided with evidence-based medicine. Since becoming a medical home the managing director of IMGH has been urging all the physicians to be more mindful of the imaging and laboratory protocols that would limit total the number of tests patients receive. The practice has also been working towards creating a formulary that would significantly limit the prescription choices available. Both of these initiatives have the potential to monetarily benefit the practice since all savings gained in this initiative would be split between the practice and health plan.

Dr. Smith is an internist with IMGH who sees hypertensive patients. The most recent treatment protocol suggests putting all new hypertensive patients on a diuretic along with a strict diet and exercise. For a number of reasons, Dr. Smith likes to start this patient population on an ace inhibitor bypassing the diuretic. However, the EHR specifically states that all newly identified hypertensive patients in general should receive a diuretic. Dr. Smith knows that an ace inhibitor will cost the patient a significant amount of money but and has fewer side effects than the generic diuretic. He also knows that a report will eventually be generated alerting the group of this practice and is mindful that his choices could have financial consequences. Thus he falsely checks the box indicating that he prescribed a diuretic and hand-writes a prescription for the inhibitor. His last patient mentions something about this being a top-tier drug with a $75 co-pay and Dr. Smith mumbles something about the years of school it takes to be a doctor. The patient doesn't say anything else.

Questions:

1. Should a physician have the freedom to prescribe drugs and/or request imaging and/or laboratory tests regardless of practice guidelines? Why or why not?
2. Should a patient's prescription drug plan influence a physician's choice? Why or why not?
3. When should EHR restrict physicians' prescription writing? When should there be built-in flexibility to accommodate physician choice?
4. To what extent should financial gains influence a practice?

Case 10: Whistleblowing in a Small Town

Relevant Professions: Nursing, Medicine, Dentistry, Dental Hygiene, Dental Assistant

Issues: Whistleblowing, Civil disobedience, Moral distress, Moral courage.

Why this is important: Patients, and increasingly hospitals expect nurses to act as patient advocates. But this is not always easy to do and many nurses have been punished as whistleblowers in the past.

The case: Bonneville County Hospital sits in the county seat and serves two rural Texas counties. The hospital board of directors includes the county sheriff, the head of the water board, the chief of medicine, as well as local ranchers. The chief of medicine, Dr. Geffers relocated to Bonneville a year ago from outside the state and was immediately observed breaking rules, cutting corners and selling nutritional supplements to patients. When one of the nurses brought it up with one of the local doctors she was told to figure out a way to ignore it. As long as he wasn't harming patients he'd be just fine. In April, a couple of nurses personally witnessed Dr. Geffers writing orders for bypass surgery on an 85 year old man who had Stage III liver cancer. One of the nurses took this to another physician who was able to avert the surgery.

Shortly thereafter two nurses, Michelle Ryder and Gail Fuller filed a formal complaint with the Texas Medical Board (TMB) alleging that Dr. Archibald Geffers violated the Medical Practice Act. Specifically they cited nine different instances where Dr. Geffers displayed poor medical judgment and decision making, failed to maintain adequate medical records, overbilled, improperly coded, and prescribed non-therapeutic treatments. Shortly after Dr. Geffer was notified of the complains both nurses were terminated by the hospital and arrested and charged with misuse of official, protected medical information in reporting the physician, a third degree felony.

At the conclusion of the criminal trial, Michelle Ryder was found not guilty. Charges against Gail Fuller were dismissed right before her trial was to begin. The full Medical Board complaint against Geffers also alleged unprofessional conduct of witness intimidation in that he sought the assistance of the County sheriff in identifying who had reported him, and then filed a harassment complaint against them.

(This case is based on a true case in Texas. In the real case, the Texas Nurses Association gave the two nurses—named Mitchell and Galle—the President's Award in recognition of their moral courage, and acknowledging their personal sacrifices in protecting a nurse's right and legal duty to advocate for patient safety.)

Questions:

1. What is the nurse's ethical responsibility when working with a physician who exhibits inappropriate medical practices?
2. What is the physician's ethical response when nurses confront him about questionable medical practice?
3. Discuss the reasons healthcare providers make poor choices. Discuss the reasons why people are reluctant to report bad behavior and the measures that should be put in place to address this reluctance.

Case 11: Managing Patient's Health Information from the Internet

Relevant Professions: Medicine, Nursing, Social Work, Dentistry

Issues: Disruptive patients, Alternative medicine, Internet information.

Why this is Important: There is more competition for medical knowledge coming from the internet than in the days before the internet (which was also when patients questioned medical authority less). How do we handle patients who see themselves as open-minded to new ideas and skeptical of authority, but are sometimes dangerously gullible? Is there ever a point where we don't want them in our practice? Can we ethically refuse to see them or is it unethical to 'fire' patients?

The case: Juanita is a 30 year old Hispanic woman who has poorly controlled diabetes. She is treated at the Good Neighborhood Clinic by Dr. Smith and has weekly appointments with Georgiana Jones, an RN and diabetic educator. Georgiana is working with Juanita and others like her to help manage diet, glucose monitoring and insulin management.

In her spare time Juanita enjoys searching the internet for information on diabetes management and general health. She recently found an article suggesting that dieting was not an effective way to control diabetes. This information, most of it written by physicians, advocated eating saturated fat, especially coconut oil. At her next group education session she brings up the article and tells the other members of the group that all this emphasis on diet is a myth. The group quickly focuses its attention on this fact and Georgina politely tells the group that not everything they read is necessarily good advice.

At the next weekly meeting Georgina quickly notices that about half of the class is absent. She brings this up with Dr. Smith as well as the clinic administrator, both whom urge her to tell the group that the article was pure rubbish. Your primary concern at this point is the damage this will do to your relationship with Juanita, who despite the article is finally beginning to take her diabetes management serious.

Discussion Questions:

1. How should healthcare providers deal with patients who get erroneous health information from the internet?
2. How can healthcare providers best educate their patients on available resources?
3. What are the possible consequences of confronting Juanita about the article? What are the benefits? What if you discover she has also read about "the dangers" of immunizations and dental fillings?

Case 12: Sandy's Case

Relevant Professions: Clinical Social Work, Nursing, Medicine, Health Informatics

Issues: Discharge planning, Clinical research, Authorship credit, Intellectual property, Plagiarism, Power differentials and Institutional roles.

Why this is Important: This case brings together two interprofessional topics, the use of electronic records to make care plans more effective or less costly and issues of who deserves credit for clinical innovations. Authorship at least has clear rules about who deserves credit, but it is less clear who gets credit and if anyone should gain financial benefit from improvements in hospital processes. Attention is needed to prevent the injustice of having people get more credit than others due to their role in the institution, denying it to people lower on the 'totem pole.'

The case: Sandy recently received her MSW and is currently working on a cardiac unit in a large academic medical center. She recently developed an elaborate process for discharge planning that provides paper handouts for patients to take home with them about medications, diet, exercise and other management issues. These materials allow patients to adopt sound cardiac management activities into their daily lives and has the potential to avert many problems that often bring patients back into the ER or hospital. She would like to further develop this material into an interactive smartphone app to give to patients when they are discharged.

Dr. Sam is a new faculty member at the hospital having recently completed an internal medicine residency. He heard about this program from one of his patients and asks Sandy if he can review it. Flattered, she gives him a copy of her notebook and patient handouts. He immediately sees the value and takes it to the University's IT department where he consults with Dr. George, an informatics researcher. Together, they develop an interactive IT application. In order to more fully develop and test it they submitted a grant proposal to a new NIH center for Patient Centered Outcomes Research Institute.

Drs. Sam and George ask Hazel, the nurse supervisor to work with them on the testing the application with patients on her floor. Hazel is completing her Doctoral in Nursing Practice (DNP) and the timing is excellent since she needs to complete a capstone project.

A month later Sandy meets Sam on the unit and asks him what he thought of her teaching modules. He states the content is very good and mentions working with the IT department at the university on developing it into an app. Sandy is excited and mentions that developing an app was her initial plan. Sandy is thrilled that Dr. Sam spoke so highly of her work.

Questions:

1. How do you decide who gets due credit in collaborative efforts? What kind of role did Sandy and Sam and George each have in developing the ideas? Is that

accurately expressed in the outcome of the case? If not, why is Sandy said to be happy with the outcome?

2. What do you suppose are some of the underlying reasons why Dr. Sam developed Sandy's work without her permission?
3. Hazel, the nurse supervisor also gets some advantage from working on Sandy's idea. What does she owe to Sandy, and do their different professional roles in the institution contribute to both not seeing the situation objectively?
4. When a project benefits a population should it matter who gets the credit? Why or why not?
5. Should Sandy only get credit if she asks for it? How can situations like this be avoided in the future?

Case 13: Disasters: Who Gets Priority?

Relevant Professions: Public Health, Medicine, Nursing

Issues: Natural disaster planning, Triage.

Why this is important: Good planning is difficult in the midst of an emergency, which is why emergency planning is a key element of public health policy. This case presents advance planning ideas that have been proposed and approved, but are not widely known. Advance planning is especially important as the incidence of natural disasters is likely to increase due to global climate change.

The case: A major hurricane in the Gulf hits a large city. All major services are disrupted. Power and water are unavailable and the main thoroughfares are impassable. The city's disaster management team assembles and initiates its emergency plan. Fifty miles away, the small rural town of Malinche loses service of all its basic needs and is accessible only by helicopter. Due to the dramatic damage to the region and lingering storms the helicopter was utilized for salvageable human life. Teams needed to be established immediately to stabilize the Malinche community for at least two weeks post storm.

The temperature is in the 90s during the day and low 80s at night. There is a huge mosquito infestation and continued rain is forecast. Malinche has no electricity, running water or health services. Most of its population is assembled at the High School where town leaders have created a shelter powered by generators. Everyone has brought whatever they had to contribute and food and supplies are rationed. There are still some people stranded in their homes including families with small children and some elderly. The mayor has a satellite phone that has been used for communication. You are part of a team that consists of a paramedic, a nurse, an MD, and a public health professional. You will be initiating a windshield survey of the town and will have boat access to move any who must be evacuated immediately. The Mayor calls and implores you to first treat his wife who sustained a broken arm when she fell over some debris. Another call alerts you to a house full of young children whose parents have been reported missing. The team also learns about a potential oil spill. A pack of hungry dogs are roaming the town.

Your team sets priorities for allocating limited resources of food, water, fuel, and medical care. It focuses on three immediate needs: (1) assessing health and nutritional status to identify those in greatest need of medical services, (2) identifying the most pressing disease-related risk factors to prevent further threats to the health of the sheltered population, and (3) coordinating elected officials, law enforcement and the health professionals on site to insure collaboration and teamwork.

Questions:

1. How do you decide whom to treat first?
2. The U.S. Centers of Disease Control supports a further condition that caregivers and those on the provider side be given special protection to ensure their ability to meet the needs of the larger community. Does this priority conflict with a commitment to equitable treatment?
3. How do the Red Crescent and Red Cross policy statements on ethics for disaster response teams reconcile the needs of caregivers with the needs of the community?

Case 14: Planning During a Pandemic: Does Social Worth Count?

Relevant Professions: Public Health, Medicine, Nursing

Issues: Emergency planning, Plagues, Epidemics, Pandemics, Triage.

Why this is important: In emergencies that involve thousands (or tens of thousands) of lives at risk, planning in advance can help make decision-making more ethical. It is not clear who should make policy decisions (e.g. health care workers, health care administrators, drug manufacturers) or how recommendations are influenced by the various stakeholders.

The case: There are extensive plans in place for dealing with a potential pandemic, such as the H1N1 virus. Federal and state officials in the U.S. have emergency powers that will enable them to prioritize vaccine distribution and impose measures, such as business closures and quarantines. When it comes to dealing with a pandemic, the U.S. Centers for Disease Control and Prevention (CDC) have issued guidelines that radically alter allocation principles in favor of preserving social functioning:

> In ordinary circumstances, the distribution criterion, 'to each according to his or her social worth,' is not morally acceptable. However, in planning for a pandemic where the primary objective is to preserve the function of society, it is necessary to identify certain individuals and groups of persons as 'key' to the preservation of society and to accord to them a high priority for the distribution of certain goods such as vaccines and antiviral drugs.

Identification of key individuals for this purpose must be recognized for what it is: it is a social worth criterion and its use is justified in these limited circumstances. Care must be taken to avoid extension of the evaluation of social worth to other attributes that are not morally relevant. (CDC)

These concerns seem to ignore the usual rule of rescue, where the imperatives of treatment for identifiable individuals overcome objections from opportunity costs in an emergency, as well as concern for the most vulnerable, those in greatest need, or those with the best prospects of survival. You have been asked to serve on a federal task force examining how best to distribute the H1N1 vaccine in the event of a pandemic.

Questions:

1. Who should be given priority when distributing vaccinations during a pandemic? Why?
2. Would your answer be different if there was an outbreak of disease rather than a pandemic?
3. What are the benefits, burdens, and harms of these allocation decisions to the various populations?
4. Consider the justification behind the proposed principle of social worth. Do the circumstances warrant the government's imposition of this priority? What are the dangers in such a policy? Has the principle of social worth led to abuses of authority in the past? Would different professions advocate for different principles?

Case 15: Access to Sugary Drinks: A Tale of Public Policy

Relevant Professions: Public Health, Medicine, Nursing, Dentistry

Issues: Diabetes and metabolic syndrome, School policy.

Why this is important: Diabetes is a major health problem in the US. Proposed ways to reduce diabetes rates are very important, but often raise the issue of the conflict between freedom of choice versus the greatest good for the greatest number.

The case: An Arlen Independent School District (AISD) Board Meeting is scheduled to vote on a controversial issue: whether to ban all sugary drinks from high school grounds. Three experts are called into provide testimony.

By now, the connection between high consumption of sugary drinks and weight gain was viewed as conclusive by most Members. The weight of evidence also pointed to heightened risk of obesity and Type II diabetes among high, daily consumers. Soda machines had already been removed from all of the primary grades by letting their contracts lapse with distributors. High Schools were different, since more was at stake financially and energy and sport drinks replaced soda as the drink of choice among students. Moreover, high school students were approaching adulthood and legally permitted to drop out at 15. And yet, the political trend in Colorado was toward some kind of action; it was named the thinnest state in the Union in 2001 and saw its reputation threatened as the newest cohort of teens weighed in. Opponents to any Board action to restrict access had maneuvered to have the strongest form among the proponents' measures—a ban—put on the agenda for an up or down vote. Consideration of any substitutes would be post-poned until after the pending School Board election.

The first expert was Daniel Litt, an exercise physiologist with the state's Department of Parks and Recreation. He addressed what many viewed as an unintended consequence. If sugary drinks were banned on school grounds without exception, then sports programs would have a very difficult time addressing dehydration in Arlen's altitude, especially during spring and fall seasons when high temperatures made this problem a deadly serious one. He believed that the solution for obesity prevention was to mandate participation in sports for all students. He also reminded Members that income from drink sales and vending machine fran-chises were a key revenue source for keeping sports and physical education pro-grams alive in rural areas.

Donna Decelle an epidemiologist from the University Medical Center spoke next. She cited recent data on the average ingestion rates: sugary drinks were the number one source of calories in this age cohort's diet, responsible for more than half of all the added sugar they consumed. She argued in favor of the ban to protect these children from the dangers that sugary drinks pose to their future health. She had no confidence in the effectiveness of measures short of eliminating access for anyone under 18, as had been done with alcohol and tobacco. She also cited some experimental evidence suggesting that high sugar consumption was addictive.

Burt Redine, health economist with the Federal Reserve, advanced an argument for a substitute motion. He believed that banning was too expensive to implement and enforce. The simplest alternative was to raise the price of drinks to a level that would discourage consumption. His calculations pointed to a doubling of the price as the right value. He thought that the higher price would be an effective signal to young consumers that their sugar intake needed to be rationed. He pointed out that this had worked quite well with tobacco sales and would translate easily to the vending machines without jeopardizing existing contracts with drink distributors.

In an unusual move, the Mayor of Arlen, Sophia Villarreal, requested time as an expert. She pointed out that the opinion polls were against this ban and counseled the elected Board Members to heed the views of their constituents. She drew some applause when she stated that the way to get children to make responsible choices was to give them guidance and then opportunities to make the right choices. She was not averse to posting information or warnings if the science was there, but thought that more aggressive intervention was both misguided and inconsistent with community norms and values.

Questions:

1. What ethical arguments is each of the experts making?
2. What are the pros and cons of each of these arguments?
3. How should this case best be resolved?

Case 16: The Duty to Report a Colleague

Relevant Professions: Dentistry, Nursing, Dental Hygiene, Dental Assistant

Issues: Professionalism, Duty to report, Referring patients to specialists.

Why this is important: Reporting colleagues is an accepted practice in hospital settings, but it is less clear whether and when to report a private provider. The potential risk is greater if the person reporting is also a direct employee of the person being reported. This can happen in any private practice, whether a doctor's office or a dentist's office.

The Case: Dr. Meyer, a general dentist employed full-time at the Good Friend Community Health Center, has for many years referred patients needing extraction of impacted third molars to Dr. Holtman, a specialist in oral and maxillofacial surgery. Dr. Holtman is well respected throughout the community for his impeccable quality and his compassionate care of patients. Dr. Holtman has consistently relied on his nurse anesthetist for sedation and anesthesia for those oral and maxillofacial patients needing this. Further, he is aided by a dental assistant during all surgeries.

Over the past several months, Dr. Meyer has become aware of some disturbing reports about Dr. Holtman and his erratic behavior. For example, one patient told Dr. Meyer that Dr. Holtman "lost his temper" during his extraction and threw instruments at the wall while shouting insults at his dental assistant. This wasn't the first time a patient of his mentioned Dr. Holtman's unprofessional behavior. Further, at a recent meeting of general community dentist, a colleague wondered out loud whether Dr. Holtman's quality of treatment was "slipping": he too had been hearing stories of bad behavior.

Dr. Meyer is disturbed about the things he is hearing, but observes that the results of Dr. Holtman's patient care are still very good. Dr. Meyer wonders about the potential damage to Dr. Holtman's reputation; he also wonders whether he should discontinue referring patients to Dr. Holtman.

Questions:

1. What responsibility, if any, does Dr. Meyer have to report Dr. Holtman? Why?
2. What professional obligation(s) inform your decision?
3. What is the best course of action in this case?

4. In general, how should a general practitioner decide which specialist to use? Think of the possible ethical problems inherent in making referrals.

Case 17: Expanding the Scope of Practice: The Tale of Michael Logan

Relevant Professions: Nursing, Dental Assistant, Medical, Physician Assistant

Issues: Access to care; Socio-economically disadvantaged patients.

Why this is important: While unequal access to care is commonly understood in medicine, it is less often recognized in dental ethics. Yet the problem of access is just as great for dentistry.

The Case: The Logan family lives in rural King County where they have a small piece of land that they farm. There is a small health clinic in the county seat which is almost 2 h away by car. The clinic is staffed by a nurse practitioner; a dentist from a neighboring county visits monthly. The Logan's have seven children ranging from 6 months to thirteen years of age. The family seldom drives the long distance to the health clinic and receives its health care mainly through the county school. The school nurse Ms. Evans recently evaluated nine-year-old Michael Logan, and noted an elevated fever and some swelling (about 3 cm length; hard or fluctuant) in the lower left submandibular lymph nodes. When she looked into his mouth using a pen-light, she noticed that a lower left "adult" molar had a large cavity and that the gums were swollen and purulent.

Ms. Evans knows that the Logan's are a low- income family and that driving to the health clinic is a drain on their limited resources. Further, she's pretty sure that the dentist won't be visiting for another 3 weeks. Ms. Evans wonders whether she could, in fact, assist by removing the molar with the instruments on hand. If in fact Michael's molar is infected, she believes that this course of action would likely reduce the pain and swelling. She can have an antibiotic sent down tomorrow to cure the infection.

Questions:

1. When, if ever, might the needs of a patient justify providing services beyond one's normal skill base and training?
2. Many rural areas lack a physician and are staffed by mid-level professionals. Does the fact that there are no MDs in King's County impact your decision?
3. To what extent should rural healthcare providers receive additional training in areas such as basic dentistry? What are the pros and cons of expanding the legally defined scope of practice?

Ethics Case 18: The Pre-Employment Physical: To Whose Benefit?

Relevant Professions: Dentistry, Dental Assistant, Medical, Physician Assistant, Nurse Practitioner

Issues: To whose benefit are pre-employment physicals and how much information does the employer deserve to know?

Why this is important: Pre-employment and other required physicals provides an opportunity to do screening for populations that don't regularly see a doctor, but the clinician may work for the company and is only looking to see if it safe for the employee to perform the job. Thus, the healthcare provider has dual loyalty to the patient and to the company, and a potential conflict-of-interest.

The Case: Red Chambers is a 35 year old man living in a small rural county. He recently got a job as a lineman at the county utility company but he must first successfully complete a physical ensuring that he is able to perform the physically demanding tasks of the position. On the medical history form he noted that he has been using "spit tobacco" daily for about fourteen years and states that he is an occasional drinker. At the end of the form is a signature line giving permission for the company to access and use all information obtained during the physical exam.

His physical is scheduled with Mike Rodriguez, a nurse practitioner who the company has brought in for the sole purpose of conducting these physicals. The exam is thorough but quick with an emphasis on his back and overall physical condition. Red's in good shape from working on the family farm and Mr. Rodriguez even made mention of his overall good health. Towards the end of the exam Red asks Mr. Rodriguez to take a look at a red lesion on the inside of his lower lip. Red states that the lesion has been there maybe for more than 6 months but he thinks the size and shape are changing a bit.

The nurse practitioner must complete several other pre-employment exams this day before returning home, 60 miles south. He a notes that there is a red spot in Red's mouth and suggests that he should quit using the tobacco. Mr. Rodriquez completes the remainder of the forms, tells Red that he has passed the exam and wishes him the best in his new position.

Questions:

1. Are pre-employment physicals primarily for the benefit of the patient or the employer?
2. How much information does an employer deserve to know about potential employees?
3. Does the patient's release imply that the company has no responsibilities to maintain the patient's privacy?
4. Does it matter who employs the health care provider? Should the company doctor have a different ethical code because their employer is the company?

5. What responsibilities, if any, does the healthcare provider have to the patient in this instance? Does it depend on whether he is a doctor or a nurse practitioner or a physician assistant?

Case 19: Who's More Deserving of the Benefit: The Individual or the Community?

Relevant Professions: Dentistry, Dental Assistant, Public Health

Issues: Allocation of scarce resources; Access to care; Cost of care.

Why this is important: Pediatric dentists are in short supply in most of the world even though many basic services can be offered at a reasonable cost. In academic health centers, researchers are always trying to do something novel and usually expensive. This case highlights the problem of choosing how to allocate a limited amount of money—whether to do a lot for one person (maybe even changing their life), or to maximize the number of people who benefit.

The Case: The Smith Family Foundation annually awards $40,000 to the State University School of Dentistry for pediatric oral health care. The funds can be used for an individual's treatment or to improve the health of the community. To access the funds individual faculty members or a department must apply to the Associate Dean of Clinics. The award criteria are loosely defined and include individuals and/or communities who are indigent or socio-economically disadvantaged. The fund is not widely publicized to faculty members, or to the school's patients.

Dr. Amenon, director of the advanced prosthodontics training program has a patient with 28 under-developed teeth including defective enamel. This young woman is 19 years of age and comes from an economically disadvantaged background. She only has $500 for treatment this year. To restore her to function and to improve her appearance, porcelain crowns should be placed on all 28 adult teeth. Through the Dental School's advanced training program, this would cost $600/tooth (or $16,800). Root canals and posts for six teeth will add another $2700 (at $450 per tooth).

Dr. Amenon would like to study this case, take photographs and then publish the results of the case study and treatment. Dr. Amenon is requesting $19,500 from the Smith Family Foundation.

Dr. Bray is a general pediatric dentist with an MPH and an appointment in the School of Public Health. He oversees the school's three community clinics that are housed in three of the community's most impoverished neighborhoods. Dental students rotate through these clinics and part of their training is to educate the community on good dental hygiene. Three students have approached Dr. Bray about developing and implementing a robust intervention aimed at preventing dental carries in babies. According to their research, approximately 42 % of all children in this community have dental carries by the time they are 11. They would like to develop an educational intervention to reverse this trend. All told, the interventions and the study of it would cost approximately $40,000, which includes the costs of hiring a part-time (25 %) pediatric dentist who would rotate in the clinics and oversee the study. Dr. Bray is requesting $40,000 from the Smith Family Foundation.

Questions:

1. You are on the Board of the Smith Family Foundation. Would you fund Dr. Amenon's proposal or Dr. Bray's proposal? Why?
2. What theories or principles might help inform you of how best to allocate this funding?

Case 20: Beyond Teeth

Relevant Professions: Dentistry, Medical, Public Health, Nursing

Issues: Scope of practice, Confidentiality.

Why these is important: All clinicians are made aware that dentistry is a part of a patient's overall medical care. The mouth is part of the body and its health is interconnected to other organ systems. But professional boundaries make it easy for doctors and dentists to ignore each other's expertise, to the detriment of patients. This case also asks whether a dentist (or any health professional) should keep important information from an interested family member.

The Case: Mrs. Jane Salazar is an 88 year old Hispanic woman who immigrated to the United States when she was 25. She worked as a home heath aid for thirty years and then stayed home to care for her grandchildren. She is in average health and suffers from hypertension and arthritis. Her physician, Dr. Marcus has worked diligently to minimize the side effects from her blood pressure medication, an ace inhibitor. Mrs. Salazar does not always take her medication, because she doesn't like the drowsiness it causes. Mrs. Salazar is a proud recipient of Medicare which pays for most of her doctor visits and drugs, but not for dental care. She has been receiving dental treatment at the Neighborhood Health Center since arriving in America.

Mrs. Salazar was brought to the Neighborhood center by her son Justin for her semi-annual dental exam. The certified dental assistant took Mrs. Salazar's vital signs including her blood pressure which she registered as 180 over 110. Upon seeing this she sought out Dr. Werner, the dentist. When Dr. Werner asked Mrs. Salazar how she was feeling, she said she thought her heart had been acting up again. She told Dr. Werner not to mention this to her son Justin since he had been under a lot of stress at work and she didn't want to trouble him with her health problems. Mrs. Salazar requested that Dr. Werner simply get on with the exam and the filling that she badly needed. Dr. Werner told Mrs. Salazar that he thought she was in no condition to undergo the exam or the filling and recommended that she see her doctor immediately. "You're being ridiculous," said Mrs. Salazar. "Let's get on with this."

Questions:

1. Should Dr. Werner consult with the patient's physician Dr. Marcus? Why or why not? When should general dentists consult with their patients' physicians?
2. Should Dr. Werner inform Justin of his mother's high blood pressure? Why or why not?
3. If Mrs. Salazar's tooth is a serious problem, should he treat it right away? What are some of the considerations in making this decision?

Case 21: Minor Children and the Poor Prognosis

Relevant Professions: Nursing, Medical, Social Work, Clinical Psychology

Issues: Rights of minors, Truth telling.

Why this is important: Pediatrics patients are assumed to be legal minors and therefore not capable of making their own medical decisions. Therefore, parental involvement is essential, but to what degree and at what age should the child's input be considered? Sometimes the patient suffering the symptoms understands what is at stake better than family members (including parents) or professional caregivers.

Case: Amy P. is an 8 year old who lives in a large city with her parents and older sister Fran. She began having unexplained bruising and fevers that her parents weren't able to successfully treat. Moreover, she was constantly fatigued and skipped her afternoon snack in favor of a nap. Her mother took her to Dr. Markel, the pediatrician who after running some blood work diagnosed Amy with acute myelogenous leukemia (AML). At the time Amy was not told the specific diagnosis, only that she had a blood infection and would have to receive treatment in the hospital. Amy's parents were reluctant to tell her that she had cancer since her grandmother recently died of the disease earlier in the year.

Amy was admitted to the hospital where she received a course of chemotherapy, resulting in a remission after 6 months. Three months later however, she relapsed. An allogenic bone marrow transplant was performed with Fran as the compatible donor. Unfortunately after several months, Amy's cancer returned. As a result, this once vibrant child spent most of her days in bed and experienced terrible nose bleeds and shortened breath.

At a recent meeting with the oncology team Amy's parents requested more chemotherapy even though her oncologist advised that further treatment would unlikely be successful. The oncologist acquiesced and provided additional experimental chemotherapy but Amy's disease progressed.

In the hospital Amy became very attached to one of her nurses Ms. Nguyen. Although usually quite cheerful, Amy began to get discouraged and depressed. One day she asked Ms. Nguyen if she could stop trying. She knew these treatments weren't working and she really wanted to go home to die.

Questions:

1. At what age should a child be told a diagnosis and by whom? Is it the same for a terminal diagnosis as other serious illnesses?
2. At what age should a child's wishes to change or end treatment be considered?
3. How can a physician maintain hope in the face of a poor prognosis?
4. What role should the nurse play in this case? How should she respond to Amy's request?
5. In pediatric research, and increasingly in pediatric medicine, children must give their "assent" beginning at age seven. How would this influence the decisions in this case?

Case 22: Disclosure of a Diagnosis: Legal and Ethic Obligations by Different Providers

Relevant Professions: Medicine, Nursing, Clinical Psychology, Social Work

Issues: Confidentiality and HIPAA.

Why this is important: Most nurses work directly or indirectly for doctors. The question is whether they have an independent ethical responsibility. In this case, the patient's wife wants information that we would normally give to a spouse and she may be asking the nurse in part out of a sense of trust that the nurse will 'do the right thing' and tell her. In some cases the law recognizes the rights of spouses, for example as surrogate decision-makers. What rights does a person have to their spouse's confidential medical information?

The case: Mr. White is a 61 year old married man, He has taught high school chemistry for his entire career at a large urban school. For the past two years Mr. White has needed to empty has bladder more and more frequently and his co-workers all joke that it's a coming of age thing. However, when Mr. White isn't able to get a good night's sleep due to his continuing bathroom trips he decides it's time to go to the doctor.

Mr. White's family practitioner referred Mr. White to Dr. Yang, an urologist. After a digital rectal exam, Dr. Yang recommended a prostate biopsy. After receiving the results, Dr. Yang informed Mr. White that he has prostate cancer and after the MRI, Mr. White is told that since it has spread into his bones it is stage IV.

Next, Dr. Yang begins to outline Mr. White's treatment options including hormonal therapy and chemotherapy. Mr. White refuses all treatment and advises Dr. Yang that he shouldn't share his diagnosis with his wife. Upon questioning Dr. Yang learns that Mr. White does not plan on sharing this information with her, or any member of his family.

The following day, Mr. White's wife calls the office and asks to speak with Dr. Yang's nurse, an old high school friend. She had noticed that her husband seemed extremely depressed and so she hoped her friend (Mr. White's nurse) could shed some light on the situation.

Questions:

1. When and under what circumstances should a married individual be allowed to keep medical information from his/her spouse?
2. What duty, if any, does a physician have to disclose a diagnosis to a patient's spouse? A patient's family?
3. Does a nurse have the same obligation or different obligation to keep information confidential? Does a nurse have to get the physician's permission to disclose information?
4. What are the risks of telling his wife about his diagnosis? To whom?

Case 23: When Professionals Disagree

Relevant Professions: Medicine, Nursing

Issues: Aggressive intervention for extremely low birth weight neonates; Parents' rights to refuse treatment; Appropriate care at community hospitals versus tertiary care hospitals.

Why this is important: All professionals work in an environment that comes to seem normal to them. Ventilators may seem to be 'extraordinary' or 'heroic' treatment on the general medical floors, but not in the ICU. Likewise, there may be different standards of care in different hospitals, or in urban versus rural towns.

The case: Bunny Monty is a 23-year old woman who is mid-way through her pregnancy. Accompanied by her husband, she was admitted to the small community hospital near her home early one morning when she developed signs of premature labor and delivery. Prior to this, Ms. Monty had undergone two prenatal check-ups by the local obstetrician, Dr. Amanda Pate, an older and well-respected general practitioner who had delivered practically every baby in the community over the past 30 years. The exact stage of her pregnancy was unknown. The labor room staff alerted Joe Nicum, a neonatal nurse practitioner, who prepared the special care nursery for the possible admission of an infant of unknown gestation. Joe was a practitioner who specialized in neonatal intensive care and had recently been employed by the hospital after moving from a large city. He quickly notified

Dr. Ballis, the pediatrician attending on call. Dr. Ballis, however, was attending to another emergency and was not available.

In the labor room, Dr. Pate explained to Ms. Monty that it was very unlikely that her infant would be delivered alive. Both she and her husband were urged to reconcile themselves to the loss of pregnancy. Within an hour, Ms. Monty delivered a very small female infant. The infant breathed spontaneously and was quickly rushed to the special care nursery. Mr. Nicum examined the tiny infant: she weighed 630 gm, was pink in color and had a heart rate of 140. No physical abnormalities were noted. From the infant's physical development, the nurse estimated its gestational age at 23–24 weeks. Based on this information, Mr. Nicum expected that the infant would be placed on respiratory support and transported to the nearest tertiary care facility 60 miles away.

Dr. Ballis was not available in person but supported continued care. Dr. Pate, however, was adamant that the infant was too small to survive and instructed Mr. Nicum to discontinue care. Mr. Nicum disagreed with Dr. Pate and asked if the parents were aware of the child's condition and chances for survival if she were to be transported. Dr. Pate said that she would go out and talk with the parents adding, "Look, these parents are just young kids getting started with their lives. They don't have the resources or know-how to take care of the kind of problems this child will encounter. They'll have more babies." As Dr. Pate went to talk to the patents she told Mr. Nicum to keep the infant comfortable and call "when its heart stops beating."

Questions:

1. How did Dr. Pate's training and experience influence her approach to this case? How did her perspective differ from that of Mr. Nicum, the nurse practitioner?
2. What effects did these differences have on their recommendations for care?
3. What are the differences, if any, between the medical and nursing professions in this case?
4. Who should be the ultimate decision-maker in this case, the parents, Mr. Nicum, or Dr. Pate?
5. What is the optimal process for making this decision?

Case 24: Multiple Providers—Who Coordinates?

Relevant Professions: Medicine, Nursing, Pharmacy, Chiropractic

Issues: Prescribing rights and responsibilities, Complementary and alternative medicine.

Why these is important: Most patients see a variety of health professionals. Many patients have at least one primary care doctor, a primary care nurse, a dentist, a dental hygienist, a pharmacist, and at least one complementary or alternative provider (such as a chiropractor, or meditation teacher, or supplement retailer, or massage therapist). The possibilities for conflicting treatments and lack of coordinated care pose many problems in clinical ethics.

The Case: Mary A's internist Dr. Wright recently prescribed an ace inhibitor to help control her high blood pressure. She began taking the new drug on a Monday and by Friday evening she was experiencing some dizziness and swelling in her face. Since Dr. Wright's office was closed for the weekend and Mary didn't think it was serious enough to burden the emergency room (or risk its high costs) she went to her local drugstore staffed by a nurse practitioner who quickly saw her. After a brief conversation the nurse practitioner decided that Mary was having an adverse reaction to the new ace inhibitor. She advised Mary to stop taking the drug, prescribed a diuretic, and instructed her to contact her physician on Monday.

Concerned that her blood pressure was not under control, Mary contacted her primary care physician Dr. Wright the following week and relayed that she had stopped taking the ace inhibitor. After a short exam, Dr. Wright prescribed a beta blocker with instructions that it too may have some slight side effects but to call if she wasn't able to tolerate it. After a week she again experienced some dizziness and a new side effect, fatigue.

Meanwhile he had a scheduled appointment with her acupuncturist, Dr. Vigil who treats her for lower back pain. During her visit she brought up the side effects of her latest blood pressure medication. Dr. Vigil said that he had had some success in treating high blood pressure and would be happy to give Mary a treatment if she were interested. At this suggestion Mary decided to stop taking the beta blocker and undergo acupuncture treatments. Dr. Vigil recommended four sessions over the next three weeks.

The following week Mary A saw her dentist, Dr. Chang for a general checkup. Per protocol Dr. Chang checked her blood pressure and saw that it was dangerously elevated. Mary revealed that she had gone off of her beta blocker because it made her dizzy and tired and that she was undergoing acupuncture treatments. She admitted that she hadn't contacted her physician because she was embarrassed.

Questions:

1. What duty does another professional have to contact a patient's Primary Care Physician (PCP)?
2. How should the dentist have addressed Mary's general medical condition?
3. What responsibility, if any, does an alternative practitioner have to work with a patient's PCP? If the answer is "none," is that an admission that they are not professionals?
4. Who can and should facilitate coordination of care? What is the patient's responsibility?

Case 25: Medical Errors at the End of Life

Relevant Professions: Medicine, Nursing, Dentistry, Pharmacy, Physician Assistant

Issues: Errors, Reporting errors, Patient safety, Advance directives.

Why these is important: Thousands of patients die every year in the US from medical errors, including errors by nurses and pharmacists. Each case can be difficult for emotional as well as legal reasons. Considering such situations in advance can help health care teams respond appropriately.

The case: Bill O'Malley is a 75 year old man with a history of congestive heart failure. Although he successfully underwent triple by-pass surgery 8 years ago after his second heart attack, his physical condition precludes any future surgeries. His physician has prescribed a daily regimen of Vasotec, an ACE inhibitor, Lasix, a blood thinner, and a statin for cholesterol. In addition, he uses oxygen in the evenings to help his breathing. Mr. O'Malley easily tires and rarely goes out anymore except to attend church. In fact, he's afraid to leave the safety of his house.

Jane O'Malley aged 73 is Bill's wife of 50 years and his primary caregiver. Their four children live out of town, yet have arranged a schedule to ensure that someone visits on a monthly basis. Bill, Jr. their eldest son was recently in town and spoke to his father about executing an advanced directive, something he's been reluctant to pursue. After this conversation, Bill, Sr. acknowledged that he was unlikely to survive another heart attack with an acceptable quality of life. Since he didn't want to be kept on artificial life support and was concerned about his family's stress, Bill agreed that an advance directive would be in everyone's best.

Two weeks later Mr. O'Malley was admitted to the emergency room with a diagnosis of ventricular arrhythmia and died as a result of a dosage error made in administering Lidocaine intravenously. In the presence of the ER registered nurse, the attending physician told the family that the patient died of cardiac arrest and they did everything possible to save the patient.

Questions:

1. Which ethical principles should the ER physicians and nurse use for guidance in this situation?
2. How does the Advance Directive affect your thinking in this case?
3. What reporting action, if any, should be taken and by whom?

Case 26: Industry Funded Research

Relevant Professions: Biomedical Sciences, Public Health, and Translational Medicine

Issue: Industry funded research, Conflicts of interest.

Why this is important: With many politicians cutting public funding of research and encouraging privatization, companies are motivated to sell their products to scientific researchers using the same methods as they use for the public: good PR. Scientists and medical researchers need to have a more sophisticated understanding of the business practices, hidden agendas, and bring their scientific skepticism to bear on many decisions in the lab.

The case: Deepak Khosla is a post-doctoral student in Dr. Susan Lopez's lab which studies the toxicology of pollutants. Dr. Khosla moved from London to the U.S. specifically to study with Dr. Lopez. Shortly after arriving, the lab began using a new re-agent that promotes the kind of chemical reactions that are instrumental to Dr. Khosla's work. The reagent was unfamiliar to Dr. Khosla and he learned that is was rarely used in the U.S. outside of industrial settings. The re-agent works with almost twice the efficiency and costs half the amount of the reagent it replaced. Dr. Khosla begins to notice that his co-workers are developing upper respiratory problems but he cannot directly attributable them to the use of the re-agent. Dr. Khosla decides to investigate the re-agent and upon closer inspection of the literature he begins to doubt its safety. Dr. Khosla seeks out Dr. Manne, an occupational health researcher in another lab. She was shocked that his lab was using the chemical because it wasn't safe, especially for pregnant women.

Asking around as quietly as possible, Dr. Khosla learns that Dr. Lopez receives quite a bit of funding from a reliable-sounding organization, "The American Council on Science and Health." On its website it says it is a "group of scientists… concerned that many important public policies related to health and the environment did not have a sound scientific basis" and they wish to debunk "junk science." Additional research reveals that the Council is funded by tobacco, oil, chemical, fast food and agribusiness industries.

Questions:

1. Who, if anyone, should Khosla inform about his findings?
2. Many labs are supported by industry. How then do you assure that the work is not tainted?
3. When a researcher comes upon safety issues, what duty does he or she have to report them to superiors?
4. What other considerations must be taken into consideration in this case?

Case 27: A Clash of Cultures

Relevant Professions: Medicine, Nursing, Social Work

Issues: Cultural competence, Patient's rights, Women's rights, Children's rights.

Why this is important: Some experts suggest that every clinician-patient interaction involves a certain degree of effort in order to understand one another and bridge any cultural gaps. This case illustrates this as the parents are requesting something that is 'never' done and is widely condemned in this country. Yet there are unconfirmed reports of it being done, and perhaps more subtle understanding would justify the practice.

The case: Mr. and Mrs. Moloto are from the Sudan and are temporarily living in the United States while Mr. Moloto completes his engineering degree at the University of Michigan. They have a young daughter, Thea, age 6, and a new infant daughter. Mrs. Moloto brings Thea to the family clinic where she has received health care services for the entire family since arriving in the U.S. and requests a modified female genital mutilation (FGM), or "female circumcision" as she calls it. Dr. Samuels, the pediatrician was outraged at the request and discussed it with the nurse, Barbara and social worker, Melinda. He emphatically stated that this request was unethical and primitive and urged the social worker to call children's protective service as he feels that the parents are endangering their daughter's health.

The nurse and social worker have both cared for Mrs. Moloto and try to convince Dr. Samuels that the parents are very concerned about their daughter's future since they plan to move back to the Sudan. They are opposed to bringing in children's protective services as they believe that the parents are responsible and that her parents are trying to do what they feel is in the best interest of their daughter. They feel that the Dr. Samuels doesn't understand the cultural issues.

Mr. and Mrs. Moloto explain to Barbara and Melinda that female circumcision is commonly done in the Sudan and the family will need to have this done or else their daughter will not be marriageable and could be forced to live as a beggar or a prostitute. They would like some version of the procedure done in this country under aseptic technique. If they return to the Sudan without it, their daughter will be subjected to a much more unsanitary and dangerous procedure with a high risk of permanent sexual dysfunction and potentially life-threatening infections.

Mrs. Moloto requests the same 'cutting' that she had, which is removal of all external genitalia including the clitoris. Almost all forms of female genital mutilation or "genital cutting" involve clitorectomy, and many also involve sewing up the labia to close off the vagina leaving only enough space for a trickle of urine and menses, making repeated infections very common and making childbirth much more dangerous.

Melinda explains that there is a highly modified minimal surgery option where there is only a small 'nick' that causes minor bleeding, sometimes called "symbolic circumcision."

Questions:

1. How should healthcare providers address requests for culturally situated procedures such as this?
2. How do you weigh the benefits and harms in a case such as this?
3. Does the patient being a child with no say in the matter influence your views?
4. Do you have an obligation to notify Child Protective Services? Why or why not?
5. What difference does it make if the procedure has no health benefits?
6. How do you reconcile the position taken by the physician with the one taken by the nurse and social worker?

Discussion of this topic can get sidetracked by a discussion of the very different (and more widespread) practice of male circumcision. If you feel it is necessary to include a comparison to that topic, here are some of the relevant additional discussion questions: Does male circumcision lead to any of the long term effects on men as female genital mutilation does to women? Does it have any positive benefits? Why are many international organizations now promoting more male circumcision?

Case 28: Surgery, Anesthesia, and Professionalism: Acute Abdomen in an Obese Patient

Relevant Professions: Medicine, Nursing

Issues: Informed Consent, Professionalism, Humor, Burn-out, Compassion Fatigue, Moral Distress.

Why this is important: Patients must consent to surgical procedures, but once they are under anesthesia and opened up, the surgeon may make discoveries and want to take action without the knowledge of the patient. Is it ethical to proceed without express consent? Additionally, when patients are under anesthesia, providers may make inappropriate comments. What recourse do other team members have when they experience this?

The Case: At 10 PM on a Saturday night Darlene, a 60 year old, obese woman, is admitted through the Emergency Department for abdominal pain accompanied by fever, nausea, and vomiting. Dr. Dwyer, the general surgeon is called and after he performs an exam he tells Darlene it is probably appendicitis. He proposes an appendectomy using a minimally invasive laparoscopic procedure involving just a few one- inch incisions.

In the pre-op area Darlene meets her nurse anesthetist, Norma, who has 10 years of experience. Norma discusses the anesthetic plan with Darlene and cautions her that because of her weight there is a chance they will need to perform an 'open' procedure if the laparoscopic procedure doesn't work. Darleen signs a general surgical consent for "a laparoscopic appendectomy and all indicated procedures."

Darleen is induced and intubated with some difficulty because of her thoracic fat pads and presternal fat deposit making passage of the tube difficult. Dr. Dwyer sees this as he is scrubbing in and remarks to Norma, "I hope you are better during surgery than during pre-op." Both Norma and the scrub nurse seemed insulted, and coldly avoid eye contact with Dr. Dwyer.

During some adjustments to the draping, Dr. Dwyer tries to lessen the tension in the room by making some funny comments about Darlene's body. He exposes one breast and flops it from one side to the other, while exclaiming "Let's drape this over her arm so we don't have to waste a gallon of betadine to cover it." Then, after placing his initial incisions, he tells Norma "Let's inflate the whale."

Dr. Dwyer finds the appendix and removes it, even though it looks normal. Then he looks around the abdomen for other possible causes of the pain, and sees what looks like a widely disseminated and very aggressive cancer. There is an ovarian mass, and what looks to be metastases to the fallopian tube and uterus. A total abdominal hysterectomy is clearly indicated, with bilateral salpingoopherectomy.

Norma speaks up and says she doesn't believe the consent covers a hysterectomy and suggests that the patient wake up and be allowed to make a decision on whether she wants the major surgery. None of the other operating room personal speak up. Dr. Dwyer says nothing at first, then testily says, "Listen, Norma, I'm sure you're a fine nurse anesthetist, but I am the only doctor here. We will do this surgery now, because it's medically necessary and furthermore it's in the patient's best interest."

Now agitated, he added, about the patient: "I can't believe she didn't know she had cancer. It was hiding under all that fat."

Questions:

1. Does a general surgical consent allow a surgeon to convert a minimally invasive procedure to an open procedure? Does it allow him to change the organs he excises if there are unexpected findings during surgery?
2. What impact does it have to say things about patients when they are unconscious? Could it harm a patient if they never know it? Could it harm anyone else in the room?
3. How do you reconcile the power imbalance between the physician and the nurse anesthetist? What if it was an anesthesiologist?
4. Might Darlene be better off having the surgery done by a gynecological cancer surgeon, even if it means waiting a few days?
5. Are we too willing to allow 'black humor,' and too sympathetic to 'overworked physicians' suffering 'burn-out' or 'compassion fatigue' who use humor to relieve their stress?

Case 29: Dying in the ICU: Is that What ICUs Are for?

Relevant Professions: Medicine, Nursing

Issues: Advance Directives, End of life medical treatment, Use or misuse of ICU.

Why this is important: By some accounts we spend nearly 25 % of our healthcare dollars on the last year of life, much of it for interventions that appear 'futile' (at least to outside observers). Furthermore, many people say they do not want to die in the hospital, and especially in the ICU, yet the system seems biased towards precisely that outcome. How can we reasonably and fairly control costs at the end of life?

The case: Fred Waller is a 63 year old man with no insurance. He has been a frequent flier in the ER because of uncontrolled hypertension and diabetes. His past medical history includes repeated hospitalizations for pancreatitis. He is in the beginning phases of renal failure and recently had his leg amputated. His current admission is for a stroke, which has left him on a ventilator in the intensive care unit (ICU). In many states he would have Medicaid, but it is not available in Texas to adults with no minor children. After starting dialysis Mr. Waller regains consciousness, however, he cannot talk since he is still intubated. Due to his underlying disease, his prognosis is not good.

Mr. Waller has never executed an advance directive and social work is still attempting to locate his family. His ICU nurse wants to discuss Mr. Waller's end of life wishes as well the appropriateness of a DNR order. His attending intensivist, Dr. Engler suggests waiting for the family to show up before having this discussion, maintaining that these decisions are better left to the attending who actually writes the orders rather than a nurse. Moreover, Dr. Engler believes that no major decisions should be made without the family's involvement. The social worker continues to leave messages, but is unsuccessful in finding any of Mr. Waller's family. On the evening of his fourth day in the hospital Mr. Waller's girlfriend and brother come to visit. The night nurses and resident on call do not feel comfortable bringing up Mr. Waller's prognosis or the need to discuss advance planning.

The following day Mr. Waller goes into a diabetic coma followed by sepsis and multi-system organ failure.

Questions:

1. When is the best time to discuss advance care planning with a patient?
2. In a hospital setting, which health care professional is best equipped to have an end of life discussion with a patient? Why are some providers better suited to have these conversations—it is the profession they belong to, or some other training or personal qualities?
3. Discuss the consequences of having an uninsured population for ethical decision-making: should we let their insurance status influence decisions?
4. What role should a patient's family have in end-of-life decision making and advance care planning? And what if no family or friends can be found?

Case 30: Dissemination of Medical Information to Minors

Relevant Professions: Medicine, Nursing, Pharmacy

Issues: Abortion, Teenagers, Mature Minors, Conscience Objections.

Why this is important: Local school boards are responsible for deciding what type of sexual education, if any, is taught in their schools. Thus, teenagers may not have the needed information to make good decisions and school health professionals may be limited as to what they can advise. Furthermore, some pharmacists maintain that they have a right to exercise their personal freedom by refusing to disseminate information and certain drugs.

The case: Abby is a 16 year old high school honors student who is completing her junior year. She postponed having sex until she met Matt, her boyfriend of 6 months who she liked and who respected her; he is a fellow Honors student. They've used condoms thanks to information their AP biology teacher Mrs. Stein casually mentioned in class, an act of mild civil disobedience since the local school board adopted an 'abstinence only' sex education curriculum. On Friday evening however, their condom broke.

On Monday morning Abby went to talk to the school nurse who, according to school policy was unable to advise Abby of her options. Thus, she told Abby to call her doctor.

After school, Abby tried to call her pediatrician but was informed that the office was closed for the remainder of the day. She called the office first thing Tuesday morning from school and when the receptionist asked her why she needed an appointment, Abby was embarrassed and said she was having sinus problems. The receptionist advised her that there were no appointments available for two weeks.

Abby reluctantly went to the nearest pharmacy after school and asked the pharmacist about her options. The pharmacist told Abby that she would need a prescription from her physician to get "Plan B" (that can work up to five days after conception by preventing implantation). Unbeknownst to Abby, a morning after pill was available over the counter, but the pharmacist didn't mention it to her, in part because of his religious beliefs as well as that she was past the recommended three days.

If Abby waits for a doctor's appointment, by then no medical abortion option would be available, only surgical abortion. That would cost $600 and require transportation and missing school.

Questions:

1. What obligations do school nurses have to disseminate reproductive health information to students? Does it matter what age the student is? Should the school board have any right to restrict medical information?
2. Would it be unprofessional or inappropriate for a teacher to discuss such personal things with a student, if asked?